The British Medical Association

FAMILY DOCTOR GUIDE *to*

PROSTATE DISORDERS

PROFESSOR DAVID KIRK

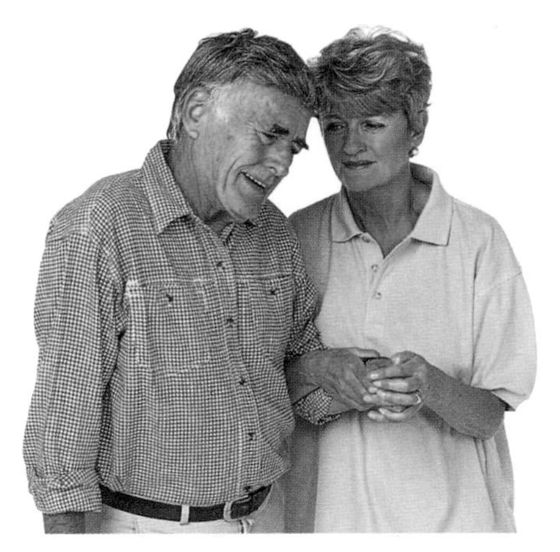

MEDICAL EDITOR
DR. TONY SMITH

DORLING KINDERSLEY
LONDON • NEW YORK • SYDNEY • M
www.dk.com

IMPORTANT

This book is not designed as a substitute for personal medical advice but as a supplement to that advice for the patient who wishes to understand more about his/her condition.

Before taking any form of treatment **YOU SHOULD ALWAYS CONSULT YOUR MEDICAL PRACTITIONER.**

In particular (without limit) you should note that advances in medical science occur rapidly and some of the information contained in this book about drugs and treatment may very soon be out of date.

PLEASE NOTE

The author regrets that he is unable to enter into correspondence with readers.

A DORLING KINDERSLEY BOOK
www.dk.com

Senior Editor Mary Lindsay
Senior Designer Sarah Hall
Production Controller Michelle Thomas

Managing Editor Stephanie Jackson
Managing Art Editor Nigel Duffield

Produced for Dorling Kindersley Limited by
Design Revolution, Queens Park Villa,
30 West Drive, Brighton, East Sussex BN2 2GE
Editorial Director Ian Whitelaw
Art Director Fiona Roberts
Editor Julie Whitaker
Designer Vanessa Good

Published in Great Britain in 1999 by
Dorling Kindersley Limited,
9 Henrietta Street, London WC2E 8PS

2 4 6 8 10 9 7 5 3 1

A CIP catalogue record for this book is available from the British Library

ISBN 07513 0680 0

Reproduced by Colourscan, Singapore
Printed in Hong Kong by Wing King Tong

Contents

Introduction

Among the platoon of characters in the much repeated British television series 'Dad's Army' was Private Godfrey, an ageing figure of fun, always looking for somewhere to 'have a run out'.

In a more recent TV series we shared the experiences of Tom, a lively elderly man, and the misery and embarrassment caused by his prostate trouble. This had a 'happy ending' as Tom enjoyed a new life after a successful prostate operation.

Situation comedies reflect real life. When these situation comedy characters first entertained us, prostate disease could be a cause of embarrassed amusement, but not really something for polite conversation. It was rarely discussed openly and seriously. The symptoms produced by prostate disorders are embarrassing.

Men, brought up to be strong guys, too often feel that illness, particularly one involving this part of the body, is degrading and something of which to be ashamed. Moreover, prostate symptoms are so common that most men will have friends similarly affected and may think it is just an inevitable and incurable part of growing old. What we saw when we watched Tom's suffering was a change in the attitude of the public, the media and, it

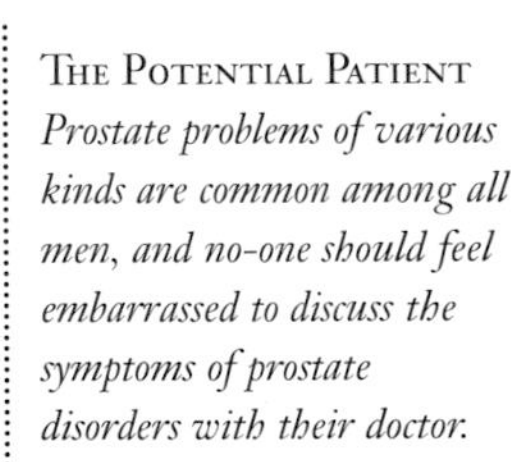

THE POTENTIAL PATIENT
Prostate problems of various kinds are common among all men, and no-one should feel embarrassed to discuss the symptoms of prostate disorders with their doctor.

must be admitted, many doctors, to this very common problem. Now, almost every newspaper and magazine prints pieces on the prostate. Famous people who have had prostate trouble queue up to be interviewed about their experiences.

The publicity surrounding the prostatic cancer of celebrities such as former President Mitterand reminds us that the prostate has a serious side. In 1997 the medical correspondent of a major daily paper underwent surgery for prostatic cancer and wrote about his experiences.

New tests are available for the early diagnosis of prostatic cancer. In the USA there are 'Prostate Cancer Awareness Weeks', and many more men are having surgery to cure early prostatic cancer. This is not yet happening in Britain, and indeed, screening for prostatic cancer is officially discouraged. Why is this? The media interest in 'cancer' has over-shadowed the important fact – that in most men prostatic symptoms do not mean life-threatening cancer. Symptoms are usually those of a benign condition, and treatment can improve quality of life. From being neglected, prostatic disorders now have become for many an unnecessary cause of worry.

Until recently, all that could be done for the most common form of prostate disease was an operation. This frightened many men and was one of the reasons that they neglected their symptoms. Now there are new treatments and, like anything new, they have been well publicised. This publicity has made many men, perhaps previously a bit afraid of what might happen to them, seek help. However, it also raised their expectations too much, and so there has been some disappointment. For many men, an operation, which need not be a fearful experience, is still the best solution.

This book explains diseases of the prostate, how they cause problems and what can be done about them. Prostatic disease is not something to fear. It is not something to be ashamed of. We want fewer Private Godfreys soldiering on (in both senses), fewer Toms suffering embarrassment and misery, but more Toms enjoying the pleasure of successful treatment.

KEY POINTS

- Men with prostate symptoms should not feel embarrassed about talking over their problem with their doctor.
- New treatments are available to improve quality of life.

The prostate and its problems

What is the prostate anyway? Most people have heard of it, but have little idea what it is for, and many people don't even know where it is. Indeed, doctors and scientists do not fully understand its functions, and there is still a lot to be learnt about the prostate and the diseases affecting it.

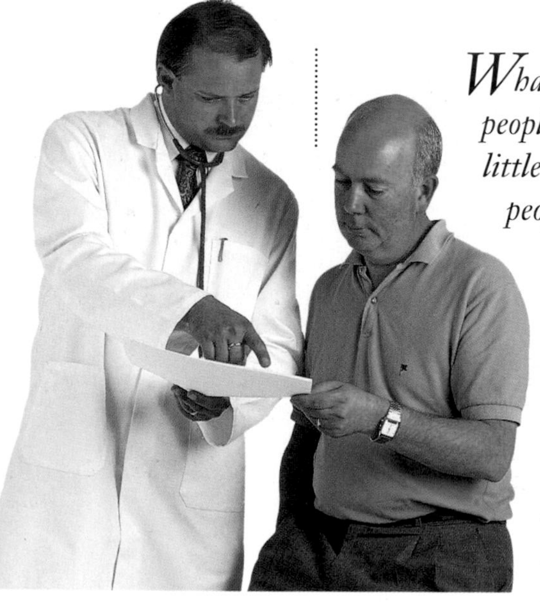

A SIGN OF AGE
The prostate of most men becomes larger, particularly after the age of 50. When the effects of this enlargement affect urination, it is time to consult a doctor.

The prostate gland is located just underneath the bladder. Glands produce fluid, and the prostate makes part of the fluid (called semen) released at the climax of the sexual act. The prostate needs hormones from the testicles so that it can work, and if these male hormones are low the prostate shrinks. The fluid from glands is made in the epithelium (layers of special cells called epithelial cells). In all glands, the epithelium is surrounded by tissue called stroma. In the prostate, this stroma contains muscle fibres, which can affect the symptoms produced by prostatic disorders. Both the epithelium and the stroma increase if the prostate

The Position of the Prostate Gland

The prostate gland lies beneath the bladder, and the urethra (carrying urine from the bladder to the opening of the penis) passes through it. The two tubes carrying semen and seminal fluid (the vas deferens) join the urethra inside the prostate.

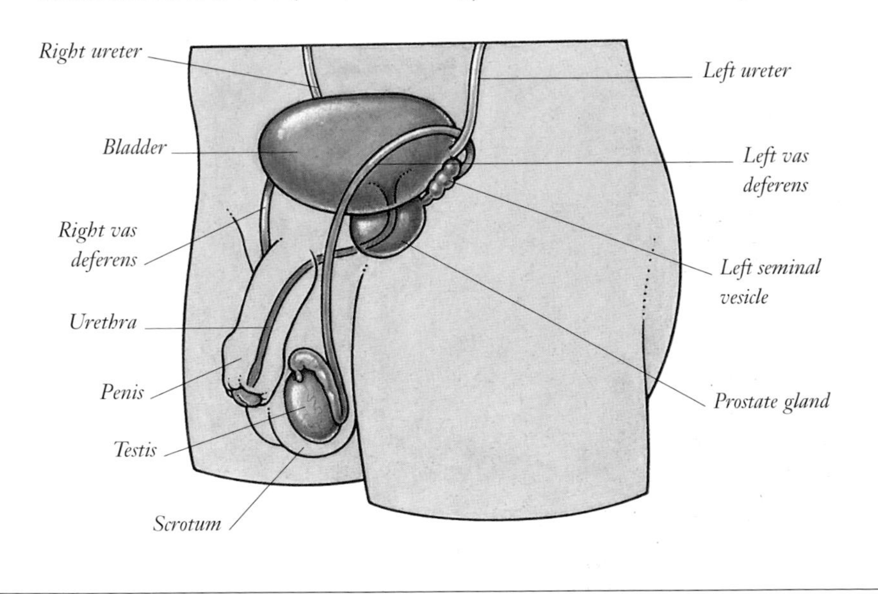

enlarges. In addition, although the prostate looks like a single organ, it really has two different parts, each of which is prone to different diseases.

Although this may seem a little complicated, it is helpful to understand the problems the prostate can cause, and how they are treated, if it is pictured as consisting of an inner and an outer part (see p.12), both of which are made up of glands (epithelium) surrounded by tissue (stroma) containing muscle.

Close to the prostate are two important muscles called sphincters. These control the bladder, stopping it leaking

Inside the Prostate Gland

As this diagram shows, the prostate gland consists of a central part and an outer layer. The two parts are affected by different diseases of the prostate.

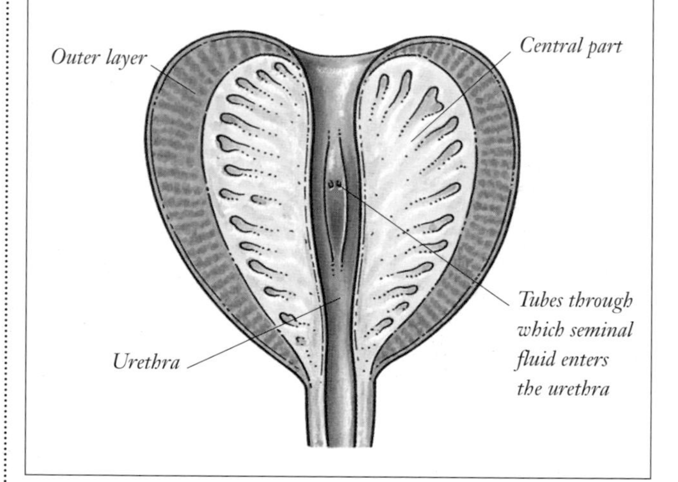

urine. They also help to expel the semen at the climax of the sexual act. The muscle below the prostate, called the external bladder sphincter, is particularly important for preventing leakage of urine from the bladder.

WHAT CAUSES THE SYMPTOMS?

As a man gets older, his prostate usually becomes larger. Most of this enlargement takes place after the age of 50, so it mainly affects older people. The fact that the prostate grows is not important in itself, and indeed the trouble it causes does not depend on its actual size. However, the prostate surrounds the tube from the bladder called the urethra and as it enlarges it squeezes the urethra and narrows the opening out of

Effects of an Enlarged Prostate

As the prostate increases in size, so it begins to squeeze the urethra, the tube through which urine must pass in order for the bladder to empty. The effect of this is to make it difficult to pass urine and empty the bladder completely.

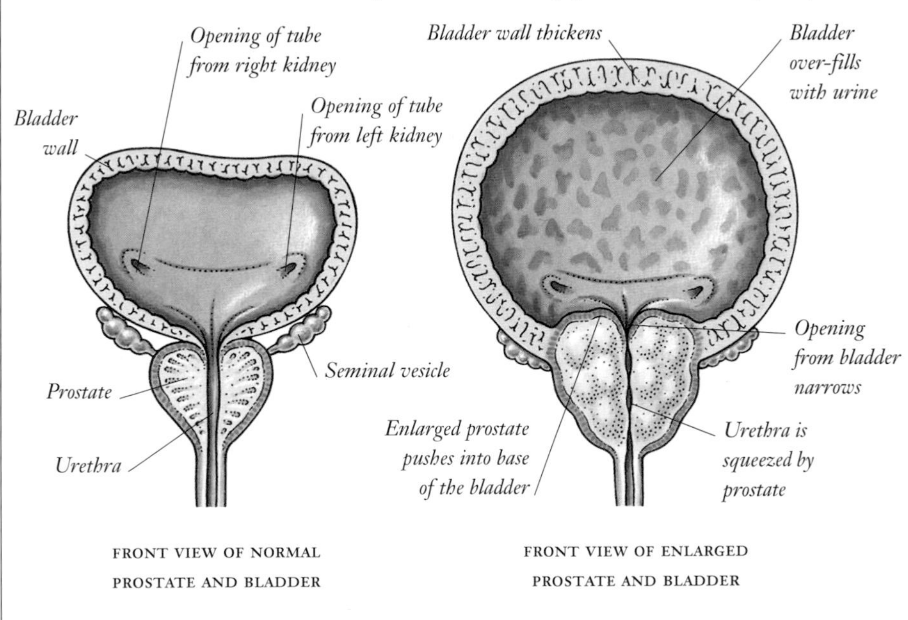

FRONT VIEW OF NORMAL PROSTATE AND BLADDER

FRONT VIEW OF ENLARGED PROSTATE AND BLADDER

the bladder. This is called obstruction and it results in slowing down of the flow of urine.

SYMPTOMS OF OBSTRUCTION

Because obstruction occurs gradually, many men do not realise it is happening. They may notice that their urine stream does not travel as far as it did when they were younger, and they may be aware that it is less forceful. As their condition becomes worse, there may be a delay in getting started (called hesitancy), and the urine

Obstructive Symptoms

When the enlargement of the prostate directly obstructs the bladder, the following symptoms are likely to be experienced.

HESITANCY	Having to wait for the urine to start flowing.
POOR STREAM	The urine flows with less force, travelling a short distance, sometimes straight down.
TERMINAL DRIBBLING	The flow of urine continues after the main stream has finished, sometimes in spurts or dribbles. Occasionally, a second large volume of urine is passed (sometimes called *pis en deux*).
INCOMPLETE EMPTYING	There is a feeling that there is still urine in the bladder after urination has finished.

stream tails off at the end, sometimes causing troublesome dribbling. There may be a feeling that there is still urine in the bladder – referred to as incomplete emptying.

HOW IRRITATIVE SYMPTOMS DEVELOP

The obstructive symptoms described above may not be too troublesome. However, the bladder has to work harder to overcome the obstruction and, after a while, this can affect the way it behaves. Some men develop irritative symptoms. They need to pass urine very often (frequency), with a feeling of getting caught short (urgency) that can become so bad that wetting occurs. If these symptoms continue during the night (nocturia), loss of sleep also becomes a problem.

This can be a great nuisance, not only to the man himself, who may have to avoid long journeys and need to plan shopping trips around the local public lavatories, but also to his family, friends and colleagues, who may not always be sympathetic.

In fact, friends and relatives are often more aware of the problem than the sufferer himself, who slowly adjusts his activities to cope with the symptoms and accepts them as part of life.

Irritative Symptoms

The effect on the bladder of having to work harder to overcome obstruction can produce the following symptoms.

FREQUENCY An abnormally short time between passing urine.

NOCTURIA Being woken in the night by the need to pass urine.

URGENCY Being unable to hold on after feeling the need to pass urine. Can lead to urine leaking (incontinence).

INCOMPLETE SENSATION With irritative symptoms, a sensation of incomplete bladder emptying sometimes occurs, even though the bladder is empty.

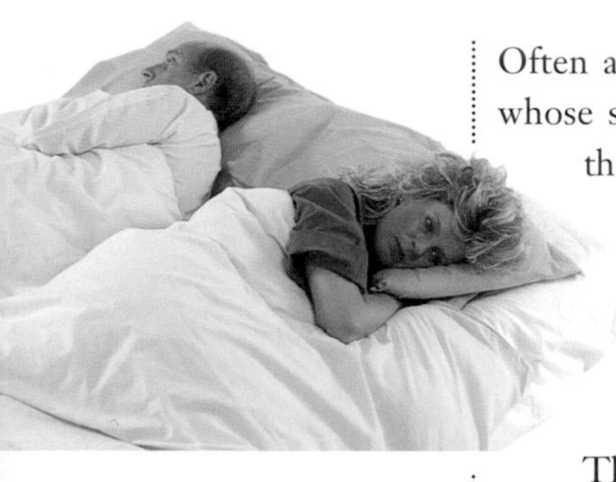

PARTNER PRESSURE
You may not notice that you are getting up more often in the night to urinate, but your partner may well find her sleep being disturbed.

Often a patient is sent to seek treatment by his wife, whose sleep is continually interrupted by his trips to the bathroom.

ACUTE RETENTION OF URINE

Sometimes a man with an enlarged prostate will quite suddenly be unable to pass urine. The bladder fills up and becomes very painful. This is called acute retention.

Sometimes there is a reason that can be identified as the cause of retention occurring. It is a common complication of surgical operations and even just being confined to bed, for example, by a chest infection, can be sufficient. Retention can be caused by constipation.

Some men develop retention if their bladders become overfull. This might occur, for example, on a long journey. Before motorways, hospitals on holiday routes plagued with traffic jams commonly admitted men with retention in the holiday season. Now we have motorways, but we still have road works and traffic jams. However, the introduction of toilets on long distance coaches has made a great difference.

Cold weather is another problem. Retention often occurs in men attending Easter weddings, when, perhaps after a few celebratory drinks, there will be the inevitable wait in the cold outside the church while the photographer is at work. Large drinks, especially alcoholic ones, may fill the bladder up unusually quickly. Drugs called diuretics, prescribed to remove excessive fluid from the body in heart or chest conditions, also sometimes cause retention.

However, retention often occurs for no apparent reason and to men who previously have not been very much bothered by their prostates – perhaps because they had the less annoying obstructive symptoms. Why this should happen is not really understood. It is possible that the final stoppage results from a slight infection or something else causing swelling of the prostate.

Chronic Retention of Urine

Painless retention (chronic retention) of urine occurs over months or years as the bladder slowly fills up until it may reach four or five times its normal size. Men are not usually aware this is happening, but sometimes the overfull bladder leaks urine, causing wetness. In a few cases, the pressure in the bladder can rise and this can damage the kidneys. This is fairly rare, but although most men with prostate disorders are very unlikely to develop kidney failure, proper treatment in the early stages will cure it completely, so it is important that tests are done to rule it out.

Other Complications

If the bladder cannot empty properly, any urine that is left in it may become infected or might form crystals that grow into bladder stones. If the urine becomes infected, it may cause a burning sensation, called 'dysuria', when it is passed.

A prostate operation may be needed for repeated infections but sometimes they are a symptom of prostatitis (see pp.75–77).

Sometimes a large prostate can bleed, but bleeding is more likely to be due to some other cause and must always be investigated. Very occasionally, repeated troublesome bleeding is a reason for operating on the prostate.

WHY THE PROSTATE ENLARGES

Most prostate enlargement is due to harmless growths of the prostate tissue, and is part of the normal ageing process. Enlargement may also be caused by prostatic cancer or an inflammation of the prostate.

BENIGN PROSTATIC HYPERPLASIA

In the majority of men the prostate enlarges as they get older. Under a microscope, this benign (simple, non-cancerous) enlargement is seen as changes called benign prostatic hyperplasia, or BPH.

The exact reason for this enlargement is uncertain, but it needs male hormones, and does not occur in men castrated at an early age. Most men over 80 years old have the condition, and about half will have some symptoms from it.

As the prostate enlarges, both the epithelium and the stroma grow (see pp.10–11). Sometimes the gland is not much bigger, and symptoms seem to be caused by the muscle in the stroma contracting, which constricts the bladder opening and urethra.

BPH starts in the inner part of the gland (see p.11) and, as it enlarges, it squashes the outer part of the gland into a fairly thin shell, then called a capsule. BPH never spreads outside the gland. However big the prostate, it remains covered by the capsule, rather like a chestnut in its shell. When a doctor examines a gland with BPH, it has a smooth surface with an even shape and feels rubbery, rather than hard. Unless it causes the sort of symptoms described earlier in this chapter, the patient himself will not notice anything unusual simply because his prostate is large and the prostate seems to function normally.

Prostatic Cancer

Cancer of the prostate most commonly affects the outer layer of the gland, but as a tumour grows and spreads to the central part, it will obstruct the urethra.

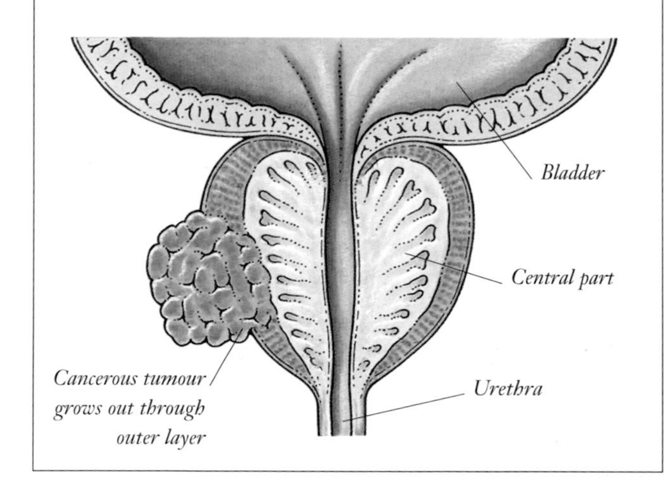

CANCER OF THE PROSTATE

The prostate is one of the organs that can develop cancerous tumours. These usually develop in the outer part of the gland (see p.11), and may not block the urethra at first. Many men with tumours also coincidently have BPH in the inner part of the gland, and often it is symptoms from this BPH that leads to the cancer being discovered. Surrounding this outer part of the gland is a thin layer of tissue, also rather confusingly called the capsule.

At first the tumour stays inside this outer capsule but, as it enlarges, it spreads through the capsule and grows into the tissue around the prostate. It may also spread by cells breaking away from it. These are trapped by the

Microscopic Image of Cancerous Prostate Tissue

In this microscope image of a tissue sample from a prostate tumour, magnified over 400 times, a mass of rapidly dividing cancerous cells can be identified by the dark nuclei of the cells, which have absorbed a purple stain applied to the tissue.

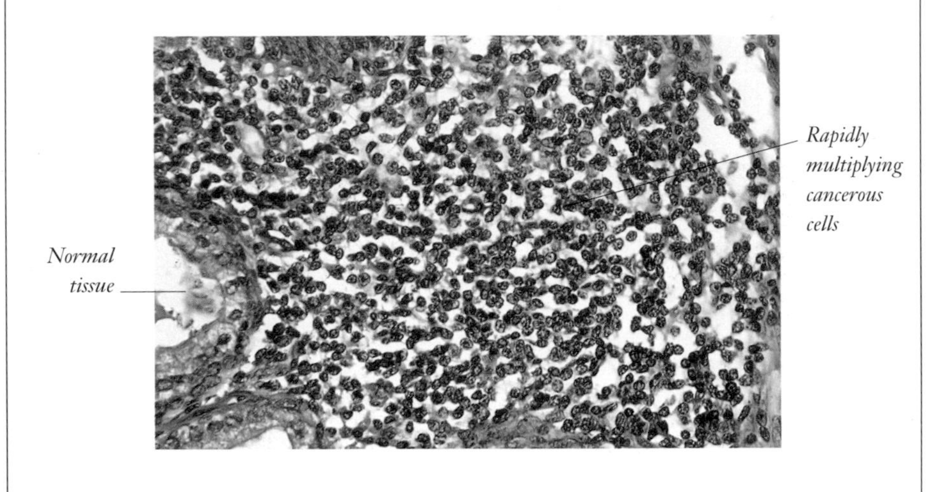

lymph glands near the prostate and here they can grow into secondary tumours (metastases). The tumour can also spread along blood vessels, usually to the bones of the back and pelvis.

A doctor will suspect a tumour if there is a hard lump in the prostate or if the whole prostate feels hard and the shape is uneven. However, very small tumours may be impossible to feel.

PROSTATITIS

Inflammation of the prostate (prostatitis) from infection or other causes is not uncommon, and can occur at most ages. Sometimes it causes symptoms like cystitis

– such as burning pain while passing urine. In older men who are already suffering from BPH, it might cause a sudden increase in prostatic symptoms.

Prostatitis may cause rather vague symptoms and can be difficult to diagnose. There is more information about prostatitis later (see pp.75–77).

KEY POINTS

- Prostate symptoms may be obstructive or irritative.
- The main disorders of the prostate are:
  Benign prostatic hyperplasia (BPH)
  Prostatic cancer
  Prostatitis.

Other conditions causing 'prostatic symptoms'

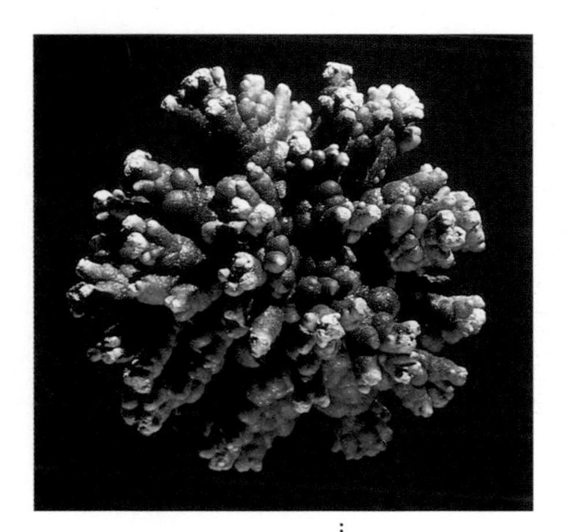

Bladder Stone
A large stone, seen here magnified, can cause an obstruction of the urinary tract, making it difficult to urinate, and producing symptoms similar to those of a prostate disorder.

Although we talk about 'prostatic symptoms', trouble with urination can be due to all sorts of things, and one reason why GPs and hospital doctors need to do special tests is to confirm that it is the prostate that is causing the trouble before advising on any possible treatment.

Obstruction

Men suffering from urethral stricture, bladder stones or bladder tumours may experience similar symptoms to those who have prostate problems.

Urethral Stricture

Apart from benign prostatic hyperplasia (BPH), the condition most likely to cause blockage is a urethral stricture, a narrowed scarred area that can occur anywhere from just below the prostate to just inside the penis.

Side View of a Urethral Stricture

A stricture of the urethra, caused by scar tissue thickening the wall of the urethra and narrowing the passageway for urine, can result from a physical injury.

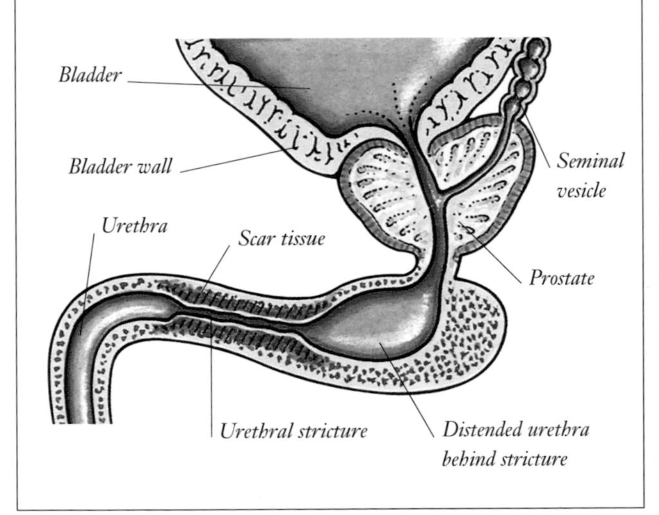

Strictures can result from injury – either from a direct blow, as in falling astride a fence or tree branch, or from a fracture of the pelvis. They can be caused by infection, including sexually transmitted disease. A common cause is having a small tube (catheter) put in the bladder – this is done as part of some operations, including heart surgery. A stricture can also happen after operations on the prostate itself.

The cause of the stricture might have occurred many years before, so think about this before a hospital visit as the doctor may ask about it. Strictures can occur at any age, so they are suspected more strongly when someone has prostatic symptoms at a younger age than usual.

Bladder Stones and Tumours

A stone in the bladder might cause a sudden blockage, either producing retention of urine, or intermittently severe symptoms. However, a stone can itself be a complication of BPH.

Very rarely, a tumour in the bladder may grow down into the prostate, but this will usually be associated with other symptoms such as bleeding.

Non-obstructive Symptoms

Real prostatic symptoms should not simply be tolerated as 'old age' but some symptoms could be due to other causes. As people get older, all their bodily functions can deteriorate and this includes the bladder. Irritative symptoms, such as frequency or urgency, are most likely to occur in this way.

One common problem is needing to pass urine in the night. This affects elderly women as much as elderly men, and many men who have prostate operations are disappointed to find that they still have to get up in the night afterwards. Older people tend to sleep less well; they pass urine because they are awake, rather than being woken by the need to pass urine. Sometimes the kidneys are not as good at restricting the amount of urine they make in the night, and some drugs increase the amount of urine.

Some diseases, like diabetes, which may start in old age, can increase urine production and will affect the number of times the bladder needs to be emptied. Some diseases of the nervous system, including strokes and Parkinson's disease, can affect the bladder.

A change in lifestyle may also cause trouble. After retiring from work, many men drink more tea or coffee than before, or visit the pub at lunchtime. More fluid in means more fluid out – and therefore they need to pass urine more often.

Trouble with your bladder does not have to be an inevitable feature of getting old. However, when it is due to the prostate, a prostate operation is not an infallible cure for every urinary symptom. Sometimes it must be avoided as it might make things worse. Before having any treatment, the condition must be properly assessed and the next chapter explains what procedures are used to do this, why they are done and what the results mean.

BLOOD IN THE URINE

It is most important that blood in the urine (haematuria) should not be considered a 'prostate symptom', because up to a third of the people seen by urologists with this symptom are found to have something potentially serious, such as a tumour in the bladder or (less often) a tumour in the kidney.

Many of these tumours are not frankly cancerous and can be cured. In all cases, the sooner they are diagnosed, the more likely they are to be cured and the easier the treatment will be.

Blood in the urine is investigated by using an X-ray procedure called an intravenous urogram (or sometimes an ultrasound scan) and a cystoscopy (see p.35). If you see blood in your urine, do not ignore it, even if it goes away. You should see your doctor straight away.

Sometimes, blood that is not visible to the naked eye is found when a urine specimen is tested. Although this is less likely to be due to something serious than visible bleeding, it is still best to have it checked out.

KEY POINTS

- Urethral strictures, bladder stones and bladder tumours can all cause 'prostatic symptoms'.
- So can deteriorating body functions associated with old age and lifestyle changes.

Having the prostate investigated

If you are a man of the right age for prostate problems, having read so far you will probably be wondering whether you need to have your prostate seen to.

Why not look at the questions in the table on p.29 – if you only have one or two of them then you do not have much of a problem and probably have no need to worry. Your GP may arrange routine health check-ups for you, especially if you are over 75, and these may include checking the prostate. If you have bad symptoms that you have been neglecting, then you certainly should do something about them.

The first thing you should do is consult your own GP. If you seem to have a prostate problem, you will usually be referred to a urologist – a surgeon who specialises not only in

SEEING THE UROLOGIST
If you are referred to a urologist, your consultation will probably begin with a general examination, including taking your blood pressure.

diseases of the prostate, but also the kidneys, the bladder and male sexual organs. The urologist will need to decide if your symptoms are caused by enlargement of the prostate, whether the enlargement is benign and what treatment if any is needed. This will involve you answering some questions, being examined and having some special tests.

SEEING A DOCTOR

Knowing about a patient's symptoms is important, not only in making the correct diagnosis, but also in deciding if and how the condition should be treated. It is a good idea to think about your symptoms carefully before you see the doctor, as this will help you to answer the questions. It is also important to tell the doctor why you are concerned about your symptoms.

Some men simply want to be reassured that their symptoms are not a sign of something serious, in which case, provided all is well, they may then not want to be offered any treatment. Other men have such uncomfortable symptoms that they are desperate to have them treated.

If you are simply worried and want reassurance, do not be afraid to say this. The doctor will not mind, and it will avoid a misunderstanding that could lead to you getting the wrong advice.

SYMPTOM QUESTIONNAIRES

The doctor may use a set of standard questions from a printed list, or may use a computer. In some hospitals you may be given the questionnaire beforehand. If this happens, someone will go through the answers and deal with anything that is not clear. The questions are

Prostate Self-assessment Questions

If your answer is 'yes' to any of these questions, then you may have a prostate problem and you should consult your GP.

Do you have difficulty in starting to pass urine?	Yes	No
Does it takes you too long to pass urine?	Yes	No
Do you pass urine in fits and starts?	Yes	No
Do you continue to dribble urine, without your full control, when you have tried to stop?	Yes	No
Are you woken up from your sleep more than twice per night by the need to pass urine?	Yes	No
Do you sometimes have to rush to the toilet to pass urine?	Yes	No

Courtesy of the Prostate Forum

designed to find out what the problem is, and how severe the symptoms are. The severity is given a number and the numbers for all the questions can then be added up to give a 'score' that measures the seriousness of the problem. Questions about your general health are also important, especially if an operation is being considered.

Having an Examination

You will need to have a general examination, including checking blood pressure, and an examination relating to the prostate. Your abdomen will be checked, making sure that your bladder is not enlarged. Your penis and testes will be examined. Sometimes narrowing of the opening in the foreskin – phimosis – can cause similar symptoms to those arising from the prostate, and a simple circumcision operation may be all that is needed.

The final part of the examination is feeling the prostate itself. This can only be done by the doctor putting his finger through your back passage into your rectum. This is called a rectal examination. You have probably heard about it, and many men get worried and anxious about it. Indeed sometimes this is why men do not admit to their prostate symptoms.

It is natural to be apprehensive about this type of examination, and the doctor realises that it is embarrassing and undignified, and will do it as discretely as possible. You should tell the doctor if you have some problem affecting your back passage – such as piles or pain when you open your bowels.

Usually you will be asked to lie on your left side, although some doctors prefer another position. It is important to relax as much as possible. Bending up your knees makes your prostate easier to feel. The doctor wears a thin soft glove on which he puts some jelly to allow the finger to slip in easily.

The examination usually only takes a few seconds, and tells the doctor how big your prostate is, and whether it is enlarged from BPH or another cause. Normally the prostate is not tender, but if prostatitis is suspected you may be asked whether touching the prostate is painful, and very occasionally the prostate may be massaged during the examination to obtain a specimen of fluid from it. The rectum itself may also be examined.

UNDERGOING TESTS

The doctor now knows what symptoms you have, how troublesome they are, what your prostate is like on examination and how fit you are. He or she will usually have a good idea what the problem is, but will want tests carried out to confirm this and to help plan your treatment. Some tests are done in nearly all cases, others only in certain situations.

You will be asked for a sample of your urine – this might be collected when the flow test is done (see below). A blood sample is usually taken to check how your kidneys are working and to measure a substance called prostate-specific antigen (PSA). PSA is so important that there is a chapter about it (see p.53). The blood test results usually take a few days to come through.

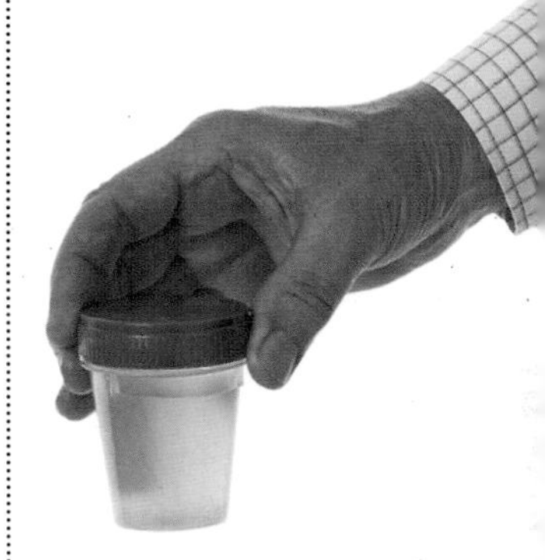

PROVIDING A SAMPLE
After your examination, the doctor will usually ask you to provide a urine sample that will be sent to the laboratory for analysis.

URINE FLOW MEASUREMENT

If the prostate obstructs the bladder opening, it will slow down the passage of urine. Machines that measure the flow of urine are used to test this. The test is very simple – you pass urine into a funnel-shaped container, just as if you were using a toilet, and all the measurements are done automatically.

However, the test is only accurate if a fairly large amount of urine is passed. It is a good idea to drink plenty of fluid before you go to the hospital and, if you can attend with your bladder comfortably full, so much the better. Do not worry if you haven't been able to do this – you will be given some water to drink and allowed

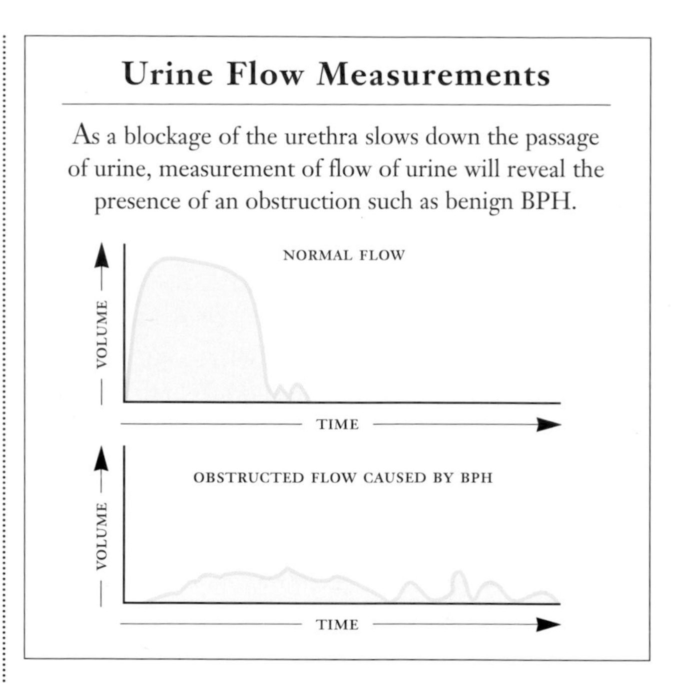

to wait until your bladder has filled before doing the test. If while you are in the waiting room you feel you need to pass urine, tell one of the clinic staff. You may be able to do the flow test straight away.

Sometimes when you first do the test you might pass only a little urine. If this happens and then a few minutes later you suddenly feel the urge to go again, do not go to the toilet, but tell one of the staff so you can use the flow machine again! When you are passing urine into the machine, relax – straining will affect the reading. Try and keep the stream in one direction; letting it 'wander' around the side may cause a false reading. You should also avoid knocking against the machine while using it. These precautions will help to produce a good record to show if the prostate is causing obstruction or not.

X-RAYS AND ULTRASOUND

Men with prostate disease used to have an X-ray called an intravenous urogram (IVU), which involved an injection of a dye so that the kidneys show up on X-ray. Now, an IVU is done only in certain circumstances – for example, if blood has been seen in your urine.

A simple X-ray of your abdomen can be useful and is particularly good at making sure that there isn't a stone in your bladder or kidneys. It also shows the size of the bladder, and so is usually done after passing urine – perhaps immediately after the flow test – to check how completely the bladder is emptying.

An ultrasound scan is used to look at the kidneys, and is very easy – a doctor or radiographer simply runs a small probe over the back and the front of your abdomen. Ultrasound can also be used to measure how well your bladder is emptying. This can be done at the same time as the kidneys are scanned, but there are also small portable machines designed just for this purpose and one of these might be used either by a doctor or a nurse in the clinic.

UNDERGOING ADDITIONAL TESTS

The tests described above will generally be done on most men with prostate trouble. In certain circumstances, other tests might be needed. As mentioned, an IVU may be done if there has been bleeding or if kidney stones are suspected, or if an abnormality is found in the kidney on an ultrasound scan.

TRANSRECTAL ULTRASOUND SCAN

A transrectal ultrasound scan is done using a metal probe that is gently passed into the rectum and allows the inside of the prostate to be looked at. If necessary, a fine needle can be passed through it into the prostate to take small pieces for microscopic examination (needle biopsy). This test will be done if an accurate measurement of the size of the prostate is needed, or if cancer is suspected. Some urology clinics have a portable machine for this test and they use it on most patients with prostate disorders.

CYSTOMETROGRAM

Fairly often an important test called a cystometrogram (or urodynamics) is needed. To do this, a small tube called a catheter is passed through the urethra to measure the pressure inside the bladder. This pressure is measured as the bladder is filled with fluid.

Sometimes this test will show spasms of increased pressure, a condition called an 'unstable bladder', which is one cause of frequency and urgency. This is one of the things that can happen when BPH obstructs the urethra, and there is a good chance that it will improve after an operation on the prostate. However, there are other reasons for having an unstable bladder, and if it is not the result of BPH, a prostate operation will not improve it and might even make the symptoms worse.

Measuring the pressure while urine is being passed is also important. A poor flow (see p. 32) is usually caused by blockage from BPH. The bladder has to work harder so the pressure in the bladder is higher than normal. However, sometimes a poor flow results not because of obstruction by the prostate, but because the bladder itself is weak – in this case the bladder pressure will be less than normal. This is another condition that will not improve after an operation on the prostate.

Sometimes the opposite might occur – the bladder will work very hard indeed, producing such a high pressure that the actual flow rate will be fairly good. Then a prostate operation is very important.

Having a cystometrogram is not very pleasant as it involves having a catheter passed into the bladder, and usually another tube is put into the back passage. You are joined up to a rather complicated looking recording machine. It is a little uncomfortable having the bladder filled up, and then passing urine with a tube still in the bladder. For this reason, it is usually only advised with prostate disorders if an operation is being considered and when results from the other simpler tests are not completely clear. It is then very important, as it avoids the wrong treatment being given.

A new method of performing a cystometrogram is being used in a few hospitals. The tubes are connected to a small portable device, attached to a belt. The patient can walk about and the measurements are done for several hours as the bladder fills and empties naturally during normal activities. This is called ambulatory urodynamics and may be used more widely in future.

CYSTOSCOPY

Examining the bladder and prostate by looking inside it with an instrument called a cystoscope is an important test in some circumstances. It is essential if there has been blood in the urine. It may be advised if symptoms are mainly of the irritative type when they might be due to some condition in the bladder itself. The urethra is also examined, so it is a good way of ruling out a urethral stricture.

Some surgeons find cystoscopy helpful in planning an operation to see what the prostate looks like first. In the past, when only rigid metal cystoscopes were available, a general anaesthetic was usually given. Now, the urologist often uses a flexible cystoscope that can be passed into the bladder with very little discomfort. A jelly containing local anaesthetic is used to numb the urethra.

The examination takes a few minutes and, because the instrument is flexible, it is even possible for the patient to see inside his own bladder! To improve the view some fluid is run in during the examination. This may feel a little cold, but will also make the bladder feel full (which it is but not with urine!). Do not worry about having an accident – you probably will not, but even so the examination area is designed to cope with a bit of water. You will be asked to pass water afterwards. If you are unable or if you feel you have not emptied your bladder properly, tell somebody – do no go home until you are comfortable.

After a cystometrogram or cystoscopy you may feel sore, have burning after passing urine, or see some blood in the urine. This settles down quickly, especially if you drink plenty for a few days. If it does not, or if you find it difficult to urinate, ring up the clinic or see your own GP.

KEY POINTS

- A prostate operation is not an infallible cure for every urinary symptom. Before treatment, the condition must be thoroughly assessed.
- The doctor will want to ask you some questions, examine you and carry out some tests to assess the cause of your symptoms.
- Some of the tests, such as cystoscopy, may cause discomfort and some blood in the urine for a day or two.

How can BPH be treated?

Until very recently, the only real treatment for BPH was an operation. If their symptoms are not too bad, most men just need reassurance that their condition is not dangerous, and advice about simple measures such as being sensible about the amount of fluid they drink, taking enough time to empty the bladder and learning to live with what may be only minor symptoms.

Why isn't treatment always given? There is always a risk of side-effects from any treatment (whether surgery or drugs) and, if the symptoms are mild, the side-effects could be worse than the condition itself. Research has shown that prostate operations are usually very successful if the patient has been suffering severe symptoms, but many men with only mild symptoms are disappointed with the result.

SIMPLE MEASURES
Taking such steps as drinking enough liquid or not drinking too much can help to improve the symptoms of BPH.

An operation remains the most effective method of

treating BPH. An operation rather than some other type of treatment is essential if the patient has had retention of urine, or obstruction has caused kidney failure. Sometimes the tests will show that the obstruction is so bad that an operation can prevent a complication of this type. If symptoms are very bad, an operation is usually the best way to improve them. Even if the symptoms are milder, when the tests have shown that the prostate is causing bad obstruction, an operation may be the only way of putting things right.

Compared with some types of surgery, prostate operations are really quite safe. Men with quite serious health problems can have a prostate operation without coming to harm, but an older or less fit man really should be having quite a lot of problems to make an operation advisable.

Whether an operation is necessary often depends very much on how badly the symptoms affect the patient. Unless there is some reason why a prostate operation is essential because of a risk to health (which is unusual), you can expect the urologist to discuss it with you and he may even leave the final choice to you.

TYPES OF OPERATION

The earliest operations on the prostate were done as 'open' surgery – removing the enlarged part of the gland through a surgical incision. Even today, if the gland is very large, this operation is still the best method and is usually very successful.

Just before the last war, urologists in America started carrying out an operation called transurethral resection of the prostate, or TURP. It was one of the earliest types of minimally invasive or 'keyhole' surgery operations, and

Performing a Transurethral Resection

A resectoscope, which is inserted through the urethra, enables the surgeon to see the enlarged prostate and then to cut away and remove the part of the gland that is causing the obstruction.

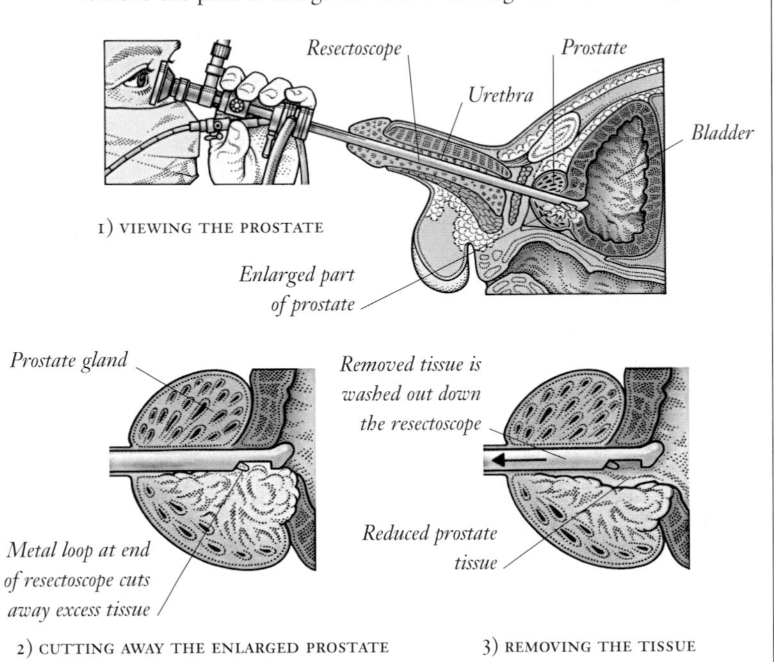

now nearly all prostate operations are done this way. An instrument called a resectoscope is passed into the prostate along the urethra. The urologist can see the prostate through it, and uses a special type of localised electric current through a metal loop to cut the prostate out in pieces. Once the enlarged prostate has been cut away, any bleeding blood vessels can be sealed, also using an electric current, leaving a cavity in the middle of the gland through which urine will pass easily.

Although the sphincter muscle around the neck of the bladder is cut away (see p.41), the surgeon will take great care not to injure the external bladder sphincter below the prostate and usually control of the urine after a TURP is good. The raw cavity left after the operation soon develops a protective lining called epithelium.

The operation usually takes about half an hour. A general anaesthetic may be used, but often the operation is done with the patient awake, but numb from the waist down under a spinal anaesthetic, given through a needle in the back. Many surgeons now use a small television camera to project a picture of the operation on a screen, and it is quite possible for the patient to watch his operation being done, but only if he wants to, of course.

If you are to have a TURP you will probably be admitted to hospital the day before. A final physical examination, some blood tests and other tests, including a chest X-ray, will be carried out. The urologist and anaesthetist will discuss the operation with you. You may be given a choice between a general and a spinal anaesthetic, although sometimes, for example if you have a bad chest disease, a general anaesthetic might not be advisable.

After the Operation

Transurethral resection requires only a brief hospital stay, usually 4–5 days. As the TURP procedure does not involve a surgical incision, postoperative pain is considerably less than in a more invasive type of surgery.

Bleeding

After the operation, a flexible tube called a catheter is put into the bladder to drain the urine; it is usually removed

The Results of a Complete Resection

Resection cuts away all of the central part of the prostate gland, removing the enlarged part of the gland, increasing the width of the urethra, and allowing the urine to flow normally.

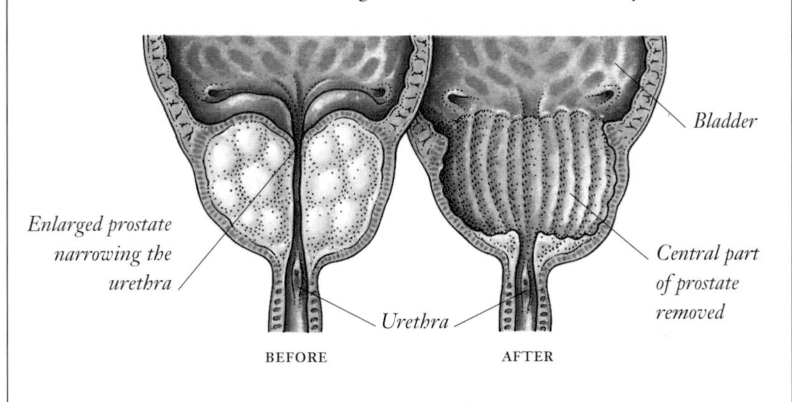

within two days. Although the urologist controls most of the bleeding at the end of the operation, some blood will drain with the urine. This can be quite bloody for a day or two. Occasionally, the blood will clot and block the catheter. If this happens a doctor or nurse will clear the clot with a syringe. Many urologists use special catheters to run fluid through the bladder to reduce the risk of clotting occurring.

Will It Be Painful?

You will not have any of the usual type of postoperative pain, but the catheter can be uncomfortable, and may make the bladder feel full. Sometimes painful spasms occur. If these are severe, drugs can be prescribed to control them. You will be asked to drink a lot of water each day to help flush out your bladder.

Returning to Normal Life

Once the catheter is removed, you should be able to pass urine almost at once. It is normal to have some frequency for a day or two, and often it is difficult to control the urine at first. A physiotherapist (or a nurse) will teach you some exercises to help control the urine. Most men go home a couple of days after the catheter is removed. Sometimes it is difficult to pass urine first of all, but persevering for a few hours usually does the trick. If not the catheter sometimes needs replacing. If this happens, do not despair – usually everything is fine when it is taken out again.

Although there is no painful incision to heal up, it is important to realise that, inside, the prostate is raw and needs time to heal. This takes a few weeks, and it is important to take it easy for this time. Continue to drink plenty of fluid (but not alcohol!). Avoid heavy lifting and don't drive for 2–3 weeks. Sexual intercourse should also be avoided for this period. You must expect to see some bits of tissue in the urine from time to time – this is like the scab coming off a skin wound and, as happens when a scab comes off, a little bleeding sometimes occurs.

Traces of blood in the urine are very common after a prostate operation. Sometimes heavier bleeding occurs, usually 1–2 weeks after the operation. Do not panic if this happens; a little blood goes a long way in the urine and often it looks worse than it is. Drink plenty, and if it does not stop in a few hours, contact your doctor.

Sometimes blood clots make it difficult to pass urine. If that happens you might need to go back into hospital, and sometimes a catheter will be put back for a day or two. Such bleeding usually settles down. Sometimes it is due to an infection, in which case antibiotics are given. Because BPH creeps up on most men unawares over some years, they are surprised by the force of their urine stream after a TURP. This usually is immediately obvious, but when frequency is the main symptom it may take longer to improve, and may not return completely to normal. Needing to pass urine in the night may persist after the operation because this symptom is often as much a feature of getting old as of actual prostate disease. The other symptom that may not improve is leakage at the end of passing urine. Indeed some men only notice this for the first time after the operation. Urine leaks out from the cavity inside the prostate. It can usually be controlled by taking a little care when passing urine.

Something that almost always happens after the operation is what doctors call 'retrograde ejaculation'. At the end of the sex act, a normal climax is felt, but nothing comes out. 'Having a dry run' describes exactly what happens. The muscle at the neck of the bladder, above the prostate, has to be removed with the prostate tissue and this means that semen leaks into the bladder rather than coming out normally. Usually, sex is otherwise unaffected, although a few men do experience difficulty in having an erection after the operation.

After a prostate operation, your control of urine should be normal. If your symptoms before the operation were of the irritative type, leakage may occur at first and you may need some tablets to calm down your bladder, often only as a temporary measure. More rarely, the lower sphincter muscle is weakened by the operation. This will usually improve with muscle strengthening exercises. It is very unusual for this to be permanent, but operations can be done to put it right if all else fails. Leakage can occasionally be due to insufficient prostate being cut away and the bladder not emptying completely. If so, a second TURP might be needed.

Men who have had a TURP are among the most satisfied customers seen in a urology clinic. The majority are delighted with the operation. A few are disappointed with the result – often those whose symptoms were fairly mild before the operation, and who find that side-effects such as those above are worse than their original symptoms.

A poor result from a TURP usually means that the operation was not the best treatment for that patient, rather than anything having gone wrong with the operation itself. That is why it is important for the right tests to be done beforehand and why the patient often must decide himself if his symptoms are worth the discomfort of an operation and the risk of side-effects. Above all, it is important to go to a urologist expecting to be given helpful advice but not necessarily to have an operation.

Drug Treatments

For men with prostate symptoms who are not badly affected, who do not want to consider surgery or are not fit enough for an operation, there is an alternative. BPH can now by treated with drugs. There are two sorts of drug – one makes the prostate smaller and the other relaxes the muscle in the prostate and bladder neck. Both types of drug can reduce the obstruction caused by the prostate sufficiently to relieve the symptoms.

Hormones

The drugs that shrink the prostate interfere with the action of the male hormone, testosterone, which is part of the cause of BPH. This reverses the condition and the prostate shrinks. Male hormones work in a different way in other organs, so this type of drug only affects the prostate and is almost completely free of side-effects.

A number of these drugs are being developed, but only one, called finasteride (Proscar), is in use at present. It is given as a single tablet once a day. It is important to realise that it may take three months or more before the prostate shrinks enough to improve the symptoms. So finasteride is prescribed as a long-term treatment – do not stop taking it after a week or two because it does not seem to be working. Although it is very safe and free from side-effects, a small number of men do experience failure of erections or other sexual difficulties. This usually improves if the drug is stopped. If sex is very important, you might feel that this treatment is not right for you – although sexual problems are more common after a TURP and then are not reversible. The other important point about finasteride is that, as soon as it is stopped, the prostate grows again very rapidly, so once it has worked keep on taking it.

Alpha-blocker Drugs

The other type of drug used for treating BPH is called an alpha-blocker. Earlier in the book (see p.11) we read that the prostate gland contains muscle. Contraction of this muscle narrows the opening of the bladder and increases any obstruction caused by BPH. Alpha-blockers relax the muscle, reduce the obstruction and so improve symptoms. These drugs, unfortunately, affect muscle in other parts of the body, especially in blood vessels, and can cause side-effects such as faintness, weakness and lethargy.

This type of drug is also used to treat high blood pressure but some of the newer ones seem to act more on the prostate than other organs and may have fewer side-effects. Their big advantage is that they do work almost immediately. At present, alfuzosin (Xatral), doxazosin (Cardura), indoramin (Doralese), prazosin (Hypovase), tamsulosin (Flomax MR) and terazosin (Hytrin) are in use and other ones will be introduced soon. They differ in how often they need to be taken, and some of them need to be built up from a small dose. Their side-effects differ, so if one is not suitable, it is worth trying another. Alpha-blockers can cause retrograde ejaculation, but this will revert to normal if the drug is stopped. Just as with hormone treatment, the rate of urinary flow is only slightly improved.

CHOICE OF DRUG

Which of these two types of drug is prescribed depends on a number of things. Some men, often those whose symptoms occur at a youngish age, do not have much actual enlargement of the prostate. For them, the action of the prostatic muscle seems to be the main cause of the obstruction and so an alpha-blocker is the best choice.

If a man with a prostate like this does need an operation, the surgeon may not have to cut away any prostate but may just make an incision in one or two places to open it up. The patient himself will not really be able to tell much difference from an ordinary TURP. Finasteride probably should be prescribed only when the prostate is definitely enlarged, and it does seem that, the bigger the prostate, the more effective it will be. As it takes some time to shrink the prostate, the patient must be prepared for the effects to occur. Trials are being conducted to see if a combination of finasteride with one of the alpha-blocker drugs can reduce this delay.

Drug treatment is usually suggested if symptoms are mild, the obstruction is not too bad and there is no reason to avoid a particular drug. Drugs may be tried in more severe cases if there are medical reasons to avoid surgery. If an operation has to be delayed, either because of a long waiting list or because it is not convenient at the time, drugs can be used for temporary help. Some men close to retirement might want to wait until they stop work to have an operation. University or school teachers, politicians or other men with fixed vacations might prefer an operation during the summer and find temporary drug treatment helpful. Occasionally the urologist might suggest trying some drug treatment first to see if it helps a particular symptom before taking the irreversible step of an operation.

Although these drugs have relieved symptoms in men for whom an operation was not appropriate, there are still many men who are best advised that they do not really need any treatment. Also, drugs should ideally only be used after the prostate has been properly assessed and the tests described earlier (see p.31) have been done. Often this still means seeing a urologist but, partly as a result of the introduction of drugs to treat BPH, many GPs are becoming more involved in treating the prostate.

OTHER TREATMENTS

A lot of publicity has been given to heat and laser treatment for BPH, so much so that patients may be disappointed when they find that they cannot have this done in their local hospital. Heat treatment, 'hypothermia' or 'thermotherapy', heats up the prostate. The treatment is given through a probe placed either in the back passage or in the urethra. Early types only warmed the prostate a little and only had a small effect, although patients' symptoms did often improve. It is now possible to heat up the prostate a lot more without affecting the surrounding organs, and the results are more promising. The effects are probably closer to those produced by drugs than by a TURP and heat treatment is unlikely to become an alternative to TURP for men with severe BPH.

Laser treatment is more like a TURP, and is an alternative way of removing the enlarged part of the prostate, or of simply cutting it open to widen it. There are a number of different ways of applying laser treatment. Although laser treatment in medicine is topical and receives much publicity, urologists are yet to agree on the best way to use lasers on the prostate or even whether it will prove to be a useful treatment in the long run. There is now a similar treatment called 'vaporisation' that uses a slight modification of the resectoscope instrument used for a TURP.

The advantage of many of these treatments is that they can be used in outpatients. However, often it is necessary for the patient to have a catheter in the bladder for several days after treatment and the long-term effects are uncertain. As they are 'new' they are not necessarily better. Although their advantages and disadvantages are becoming understood, most urologists still feel that these new treatments need more testing before they can be generally recommended. This is one reason why they are not widely available; the other is that the equipment needed is often expensive and hospitals will want to know how well the treatment works before buying it. Where such a treatment is suggested, it will probably made clear that it is 'on trial'. There is more about trials for prostate disease (see p.79).

'Stents' are short tubes, usually made of inert metal mesh, which are placed in the prostate to keep it open. They can be put in with very little disturbance often under local anaesthetic. A stent might be used in a man who is too unfit for an operation to avoid him having to be catheterised permanently. However, they can often cause long-term problems and are used less now than a few years ago.

KEY POINTS

- Surgery is the most effective way to treat BPH, and transurethral resection (TURP) is now the operation of choice.
- The benefits of surgery have to be weighed against the side-effects and possible complications.
- Drug therapy is available for men whose symptoms are mild, who do not want to consider surgery or who are not fit enough for an operation.
- The two main types of drug are those that shrink the prostate (hormones) and those that relax the muscle within the prostate (alpha-blockers).

Retention of urine

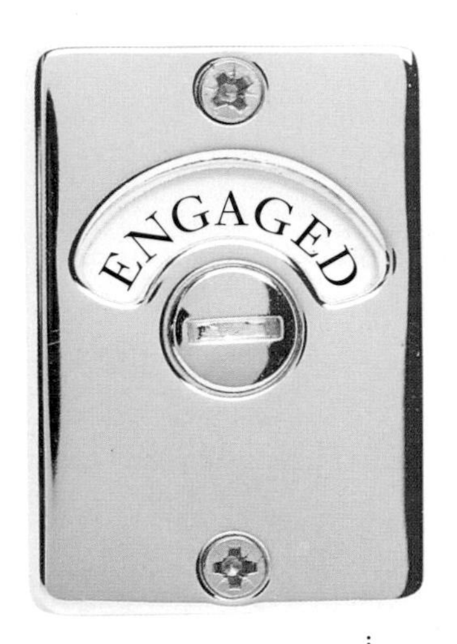

UNCOMFORTABLE DELAY
A man with an enlarged prostate may find that when he gets to the toilet he cannot pass urine at all.

The retention of urine is one of the most unpleasant things that can happen to a man with prostate trouble. He feels the need to pass urine, but when he gets to the toilet he can only force out a dribble or nothing at all.

As the bladder of a man with prostate problems fills, it becomes more and more painful. Occasionally after a long period of discomfort, something finally comes out and the condition rights itself. Often it does not, and this means a trip to hospital to have a catheter put into the bladder to drain the urine. This sounds a bit unpleasant, but it is so effective that many doctors consider it to be the most worthwhile thing they can do for a patient.

CATHETERISATION

Before the catheter is inserted, some jelly containing a local anaesthetic is put into the urethra. This numbs it and makes it slippery to help the catheter go in. After a short delay to let the anaesthetic work, the doctor passes the catheter in a sterile manner. There is usually a dodgy moment as the catheter goes through the prostate into the bladder, but then the relief is instant.

Sometimes the catheter will not pass. If this happens, a suprapubic catheter is used. This is put into the bladder through the skin of the lower abdomen under local anaesthetic. Although this sounds awful, the full bladder is so close to the skin that it really is very safe and straightforward.

Usually the patient is then kept in hospital, although it is quite possible to go home with the catheter. If the patient lives in a remote place, his GP might catheterise him at home to avoid a long and painful ambulance journey. The catheter might be taken out after a few days, particularly if there is an obvious cause for retention (such as constipation or an alcoholic binge) and quite a

How a Catheter Works

Catheterisation involves passing a tube up the penis into the bladder and inflating a small balloon to keep it in place. It sounds unpleasant, but it provides an immediate solution to an uncomfortable condition.

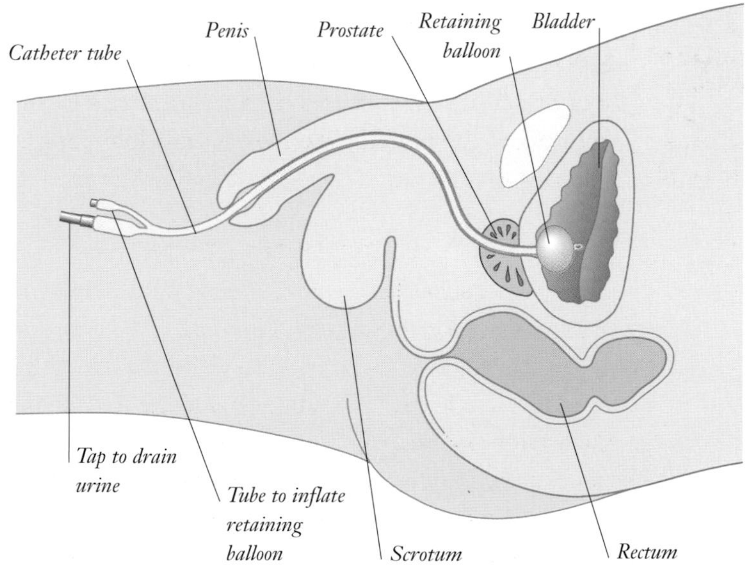

few men can then pass urine again. However, retention usually means that a prostate operation is on the horizon, and frequently it will be done as soon as there is a space available in the operating theatre.

KIDNEY FAILURE

Sometimes painless chronic retention is associated with kidney failure and in this case the treatment is a little different. A catheter is still necessary, but once the blockage is removed the kidneys start to produce copious amounts of fluid and this must be replaced.

This usually means having a drip into a vein in the arm. Before going on to have a prostate operation, the kidneys have to recover and this could take a few weeks.

RESULTS OF TREATMENT

After sudden acute retention, the results of prostate surgery are usually very good. When chronic retention is long term, the overstretched bladder may not work very well and even after a good operation will still not empty. Sometimes the bladder improves if a catheter is left in for a few weeks – this does not mean having to stay in hospital as it is quite easy to look after a catheter at home.

KEY POINTS

- Retention of urine can be relieved by insertion of a catheter into the bladder to drain the urine.
- After catheterisation for retention, a prostate operation is usually required.

Prostate-specific antigen

A fairly new blood test called prostate-specific antigen (PSA) has been given a lot of publicity as a method of early diagnosis of prostate cancer. There is more to it than that, and understanding this test and its significance is important.

Prostate-specific antigen is a substance made by only the prostate gland and is part of the fluid that the prostate adds to the semen. Some PSA gets into the blood, and this can be measured. Having PSA in the blood is normal for a man.

When a doctor does a PSA test, he wants to know how much PSA there is. Think of the PSA in the blood as if it is 'leaking' out of the prostate. More PSA will come from a large prostate than a small one, so as you get older the amount of PSA can increase as the prostate enlarges.

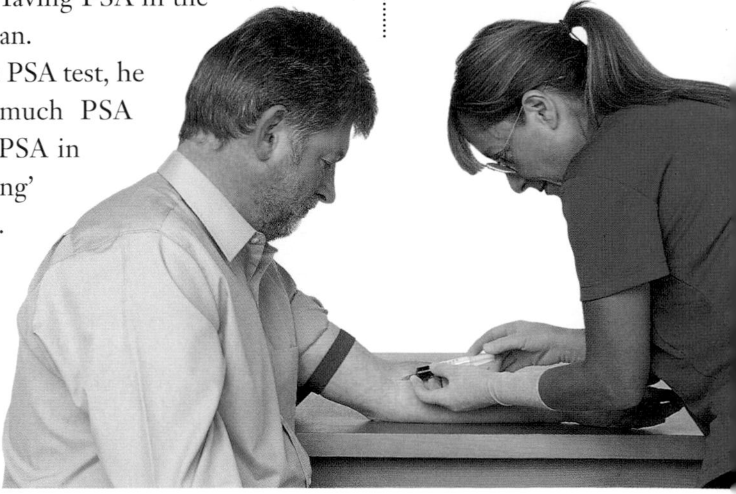

AN ACCURATE MARKER
A blood test reveals how much PSA the prostate is releasing into the bloodstream – a useful indication of what is going on in the gland.

Some diseases of the prostate make it more 'leaky' and in this case the amount of PSA is even higher. This happens with cancer of the prostate and is the reason why the test can be used to look for cancer. Other diseases of the prostate also make it more leaky, for example, the PSA may be high when the prostate is infected. It also goes up after a prostate operation, or even simply following a cystoscopy examination or having a catheter passed.

As older men have larger prostates and also more have non-cancerous diseases of the prostate such as prostatitis, the average PSA is higher in men of 75 than in men of 55. So if your PSA is higher than 'normal,' it does not mean you have cancer. You might have, but it is more likely that you have BPH, or that something else has happened to push up the amount of PSA in your blood.

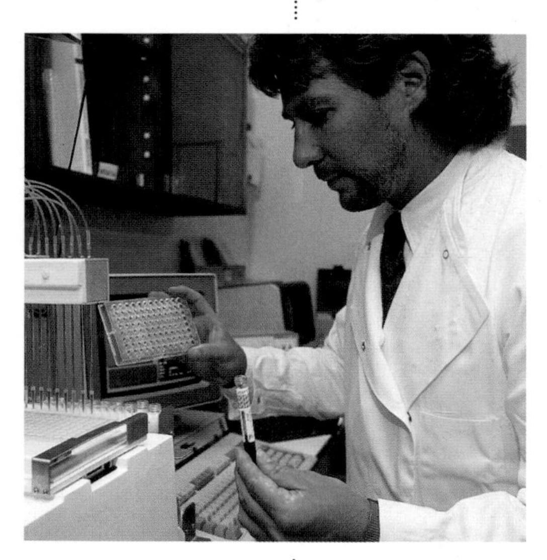

TESTING THE BLOOD
If laboratory analysis of a blood sample shows a very high level of PSA, it is likely to indicate cancer of the prostate.

As a test for cancer, PSA is helpful but the results have to be interpreted carefully. In technical terms, it is not very specific and it gives a lot of false positives – results that seem to indicate cancer but that on further investigation do not. If PSA is very high, this does usually mean there is cancer. If it is only a little bit raised, the size of the prostate and any other conditions affecting the prostate must be taken into account. It will certainly be necessary to do more tests before cancer can be diagnosed. The diagnosis is usually confirmed by taking some small pieces of prostate (biopsies) with a needle, usually when a transrectal ultrasound (TRUS) is done (see p.33). Sometimes this can cause infection in the urine or even the bloodstream. More importantly, the biopsy might miss the tumour, so a negative biopsy can give a false picture. This means that, even if the biopsy is negative, it is usually necessary to have further PSA checks and even another biopsy. It can be very difficult to be completely certain that a raised PSA is not caused by cancer.

PSA and Cancer

In a man who is found to have cancer of the prostate, the amount of PSA is a good guide to the extent of his disease, and helps in deciding how he should be treated. If the PSA is normal (and one problem is that cancer of the prostate can have a normal PSA), or only slightly raised, it is unlikely that the tumour has spread significantly and this is reassuring. At the other extreme, a very high level of PSA is sufficient to make a diagnosis of cancer of the prostate and, in these circumstances, it is often possible to save the patient the discomfort and the delay of having further tests done and arrange for his treatment to be commenced as soon as possible. Successful treatment of cancer of the prostate will lower the PSA, and regular checks on the amount of PSA in the blood are an important part of the follow-up.

Screening Prostate Cancer

Cervical smears are used to screen for cancer of the cervix in women. Can PSA be used as a test to screen for cancer of the prostate in the same way? This is a difficult question to answer because there is no clear difference between the amount of PSA found in the blood of men with cancer and of men with simple BPH and other benign conditions.

In America it is now very popular for men to have their PSA checked once a year, and there is no doubt that this finds a lot of cancers that are not causing any symptoms. These men usually will have a radical prostatectomy (see p.60), and so it is now becoming one of the most common operations in America.

It is natural for men in Britain to wonder why screening is not done here – they may have a cancer causing no symptoms that could be cured if it was diagnosed early. The issue is very complicated, however, and urologists and cancer specialists do not yet agree.

In the first place, for every person who has cancer diagnosed in this way, many others will have to have tests done, and will experience a lot of worry waiting for the results. If cancer is found, a radical prostatectomy (or perhaps radiotherapy) will be necessary to get rid of the cancer, and this is a fairly serious operation. All this would be worthwhile if it produced a large reduction in the number of men dying from cancer of the prostate. However, some very early cancers grow slowly and in many cases might never cause harm, so it is not too clear how many lives would be saved. This is especially the case with older men, so although it might be a good idea to check the PSA in a man aged over 55, it is less likely to be done in men aged over 75.

Most specialists think it is too early to recommend screening of men without prostate symptoms, but research into the value of screening is going on. If a more specific test were found for cancer, and if ways were discovered of deciding which early cancers are dangerous, it would be easier to recommend screening. It would also easier if there were a simpler treatment than radical prostatectomy.

As a general rule, it is probably wise to measure the PSA in a man who has prostatic symptoms, as such symptoms can be due to cancer of the prostate and, if they are, they may need different treatment from that required if they were due to BPH. Because of this, most British urologists are seeing more men with prostatic cancer. The chapter on cancer describes the operation of radical prostatectomy for early cancer. Ten years ago this operation was not often done in the UK and would have received only a brief mention. It is now part of the regular treatment in many urology departments, largely because of earlier diagnosis through using the PSA test.

KEY POINTS

- The prostate-specific antigen (PSA) test is a new test for assessing prostate disease.
- Many factors other than cancer can increase the level of PSA in the blood.
- Use of the PSA test is leading to more men with prostatic cancer being treated.

Prostatic cancer

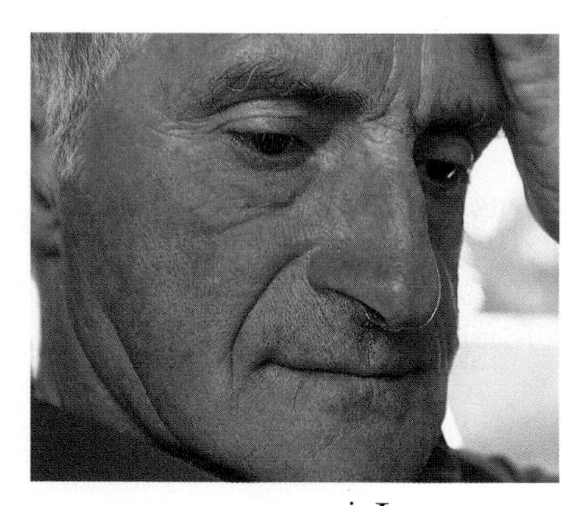

Cancer is an alarming word. Many men fear that their prostatic symptoms are caused by cancer. In most cases, this fear is unfounded, but it is true that cancer of the prostate is quite common.

THE OLDER PATIENT
In the elderly, prostatic cancer may not alter life expectancy.

Like most types of cancer, prostatic cancer can be fatal. However, it is a form of cancer for which many types of treatment are available. Also, it often grows slowly and may cause little harm, especially in very elderly men.

Recently, doctors have discovered new ways of detecting early cancers in the prostate. This means that more men with prostatic cancer are being diagnosed at an earlier stage. As I mentioned in the last chapter, there is much discussion among cancer specialists about whether these tests should be used for screening in the way that women are screened for breast and cervical cancer (see p.55).

Why cancer of the prostate is so common is not known. In most cases there is no clear family history, but there is a form of the disease that does seem to run in families. If you have had a single relative with the disease, do not worry. However, if two closely related relatives have had prostate cancer, particularly if they were young, you should get your prostate checked from time to time after you reach 50.

There are differences between races and in different parts of the world, some of which might be due to diet or environmental factors. For example, prostate cancer is uncommon in Japan, but Japanese men who live in America have a higher risk of developing it. This is probably as a result of differences in diet. Certain types of fatty food may predispose to prostate cancer, whereas other foods, possibly including soya products, are protective. It is still too early to give definite advice but, as we understand more about these differences, it may become possible to advise on diets that reduce the risk of prostate cancer. Although there was some recent concern that having a vasectomy might make cancer of the prostate more likely, most experts are now agreed that this is not so.

HOW IS IT DIAGNOSED?

The difference between cancer of the prostate and benign enlargement (BPH) is that the cancer can grow out from the prostate into the surrounding tissues and also can spread to other parts of the body (metastases), particularly to the bones, where it can cause pain or even fractures. When cancer is the cause of prostatic symptoms these can come back after treatment if the cancer grows again. Sometimes cancer in the prostate itself may not cause any symptoms, and the first sign of the disease might arise in some other part of the body.

Your doctor may suspect that there is a tumour in your prostate if it feels abnormally hard or irregular, or if your PSA level (see p.55) is particularly high. When either of these is found, the doctor will often arrange for you to have a transrectal ultrasound scan (see p.33). Sometimes the patient will need a transurethral resection (TURP) operation anyway because of the severity of his prostate symptoms. As TURP removes tissue that can be examined, it will be done promptly if cancer is suspected – as a way of clarifying the diagnosis. Sometimes cancer is not suspected, and it is only diagnosed when the tissue removed at an operation is examined by a pathologist.

X-rays or (more usually) a test called a bone scan is done to check that there has been no spread to the bones. This is done by injecting a small amount of a radioactive substance. This is taken up where the bone is active and is detected by a special scanner. This is not a specific test for cancer and uptake might be due to other conditions such as arthritis, old healed fractures and benign diseases of the bones. X-rays of the abnormal areas may help. Very occasionally, an orthopaedic surgeon might be asked to take a small piece of the bone for microscopic examination.

HOW IS IT TREATED?

Removing or destroying a cancerous growth will cure the disease, providing it has not spread. Until recently this was all that could be done for most cancers and if spread (metastases) had already occurred little more could be done. However, there are now many treatments available that can be used to destroy or shrink cancer that has spread to other parts of the body. As we will see, cancer of the prostate was one of the first types of cancer for which treatment of this type was developed.

CANCER SURGERY

Most people expect cancer to be treated by surgical removal of all or part of the organ in which it occurs, as in cancer of the breast in women, cancer of the testis, cancer of the kidney and in many other types of the

What Happens in a Radical Prostatectomy?

This operation consists of removing the whole of the prostate gland and the seminal vesicles, and then reconnecting the urethra to the bladder. This procedure is usually only performed on younger patients.

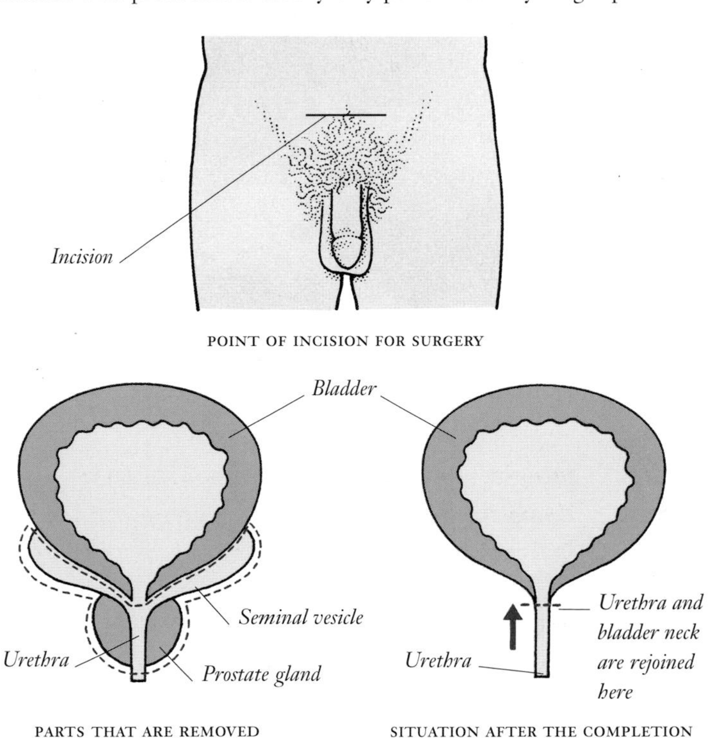

POINT OF INCISION FOR SURGERY

PARTS THAT ARE REMOVED IN A RADICAL PROSTECTOMY

SITUATION AFTER THE COMPLETION OF A RADICAL PROSTATECTOMY

disease. Although a famous urologist called Hugh Hampton Young working at The Johns Hopkins Hospital in America first described radical prostatectomy in 1905, the operation that removes the whole prostate gland is done on only a few men with cancer of the prostate. The reason that it is not common is that cancer of the prostate can be difficult to detect until it has grown outside the prostate gland. Once this has happened, it is impossible to remove all the cancer by surgery and so an operation will not cure the disease.

Although doctors can now diagnose cancers at an earlier stage, many small early cancers grow very slowly and can take as long as 10 years to cause trouble. Obviously, for a man of, say, 85 years old, this sort of tumour is not going to be dangerous and at this age he would not stand up to major surgery very well. For this reason, removing the prostate as a treatment for cancer is only done in younger patients and when there is reason to believe that the cancer is going to grow fairly quickly. Usually the operation is only recommended to men under 70, although the exact age depends on individual fitness.

RADIOTHERAPY

Radiotherapy can destroy small tumours and thus cure the cancer, so it is an alternative to radical prostatectomy. It may be suggested if the patient is not fit for an operation, and some men choose it in preference to surgery. Although removing a tumour completely by an operation may seem more satisfactory, there is no definite proof that one treatment cures the disease better than the other.

Radiotherapy can also be used when surgery is not possible because the cancer has spread outside the prostate. Here it may not 'cure' the cancer but, by shrinking it, it will prevent the cancer from causing trouble and may reduce the chances of it spreading further.

WAIT AND SEE

As many tumours are not immediately dangerous, some patients may be advised that they need no immediate treatment. This does not mean they are being neglected, and it is important that they are seen regularly, so that tests can be done to check that the cancer is not advancing. If it is, treatment might then be advised. Sometimes the tests will show that the tumour is growing so slowly that it is safe to discharge the patient from the hospital clinic, although he will be advised to keep in touch with his GP.

RADICAL PROSTATECTOMY

If treatment for cancer when it is at an early stage, and confined to the the prostate gland, is recommended, a discussion will usually take place about the choice of treatment. Because the best treatment for early cancer of the prostate is uncertain, a man with the disease should expect to be informed of the possibilities and given a major say in deciding what is done.

Radical prostatectomy involves removal of the whole prostate gland. This is different from operations for BPH, where even the open operation only takes out the inner enlarged part of the gland (see p.12). The prostate gland can be removed either through an incision in the lower abdomen or from below by an incision in front of the back passage. Either before or at the same time (possibly by a laparoscopic 'keyhole' operation), the lymph nodes (glands) at the side of the prostate will be removed and checked to make sure that there is no sign of the cancer spreading. Removal of these nodes causes no harm. If there is no cancer in them, the prostate gland is removed, cutting the urethra below the prostate and removing the prostate from the neck of the bladder, which is then stitched back onto the urethra. A catheter is left in place, usually for two weeks, while healing takes place. Most men get over the immediate effects of the operation quickly enough to go home after a few days with the catheter in, returning to hospital to have it removed.

WHAT ARE THE COMPLICATIONS?

The biggest problem during the operation is a risk of bleeding from large veins in front of the prostate – a blood transfusion sometimes is necessary if this happens. A little urine may leak from where the bladder is stitched to the urethra but this usually settles down. The two problems which can be found afterwards are poor control of the urine and sexual difficulties.

- **Poor control of urine** On p.11 the closeness of the muscle sphincters of the bladder and the prostate was described. Removing the prostate can affect these muscles. It is quite common to have some difficulty in control of urine for a day or two after the catheter is removed.

The patient will be warned of this and taught exercises to strengthen his muscles. Although most men regain control very quickly, some find that they are left with a little leakage from time to time, for example, during exercise or in bed at night, and they may sometimes need to wear a pad for protection. Very occasionally the leakage of urine is more serious. If treatment is needed, a plastic device called an 'artificial sphincter' might be put in by another operation, but this is unusual.

- **Sexual problems** The nerves needed for a man to have an erection lie close to his prostate. At one time it was thought that a radical prostatectomy almost inevitably caused a loss of erection because these nerves were cut. Surgeons now know more precisely where the nerves are, and the operation is done in such a way that damage to them is avoided if possible. However, the surgeon will warn the patient that cutting these nerves is still sometimes necessary to remove the cancer completely. Failure of erections can be treated, but usually injections into the penis are needed. Unfortunately, the new impotence drug, sildenafil (Viagra) often does not work after a radical prostatectomy.

Because nerves are easily bruised but can recover, an initial loss of erection may improve but can take many months. It is only the actual erection that is affected – normal sexual desire and ability to reach a climax and orgasm should not be affected, although there will be little in the way of fluid (ejaculate) to come out.

RADIOTHERAPY TREATMENT

Radiotherapy is administered by a machine. The patient has to lie under the machine for a few minutes for each treatment. A number of daily treatments (called 'fractions') are usually given spread over 4–6 weeks. Patients normally have radiotherapy as outpatients, although in some cases admission to hospital is advised. The period of treatment with, and time to get over, radiotherapy is very similar to the time it takes to recover after a radical prostatectomy and usually the two treatments both mean taking a couple of months off work.

WHAT ARE THE COMPLICATIONS?

It is unusual for radiotherapy treatment to cause incontinence of urine, and although failure of erection occurs quite often, it is less common than is the case after radical prostatectomy. However, because it is impossible to focus the radiotherapy entirely on the prostate, it does also temporarily affect the bladder and the rectum.

Most men will get some symptoms of cystitis (burning and frequent passage of urine) and diarrhoea during and after radiotherapy. Sometimes blood will be seen in the urine or bowel motions.

These symptoms usually settle down within a few weeks of completing the treatment. Occasionally symptoms will persist and, very rarely, the radiotherapy might produce some permanent damage to the bladder or to the bowel.

An alternative way of giving radiotherapy is by an operation in which small 'seeds' containing radioactive material are inserted into the prostate. This had become uncommon, but with improvements in the technique, interest in this method (called 'brachytherapy') is increasing again – although patients for whom it is suitable have to be very carefully chosen.

CHOICE OF TREATMENT?

Both radical prostatectomy and radiotherapy are major treatments with possible serious side-effects. It is important to realise that, in terms of risks, overall discomfort and time away from normal activities, the two are not very different.

Also, because their relative effectiveness as treatments is similar, a man with prostatic cancer should be informed about the alternatives and involved in the choice of his treatment.

Some men are happier if the tumour is removed from their body, and prefer surgery. Others do not like the idea of an operation, and choose radiotherapy. Surgery might not be safe for someone with severe bronchitis or heart disease, and he might be advised to have radiotherapy or even, in the first instance, simple observation (see p.62).

PRELIMINARY HORMONE TREATMENT

Sometimes, before radical prostatectomy or radiotherapy, a temporary period of hormone treatment (see pp.68–69) is given to reduce the size of the prostate. This is thought to improve the effectiveness of the treatment and is more often done before radiotherapy treatment rather than radical prostatectomy. During this treatment, which is usually given for three months or a little longer, the side effects of hormone treatment are experienced but, once the radiotherapy (or operation) has been completed, the hormone treatment is stopped and its effects should be reversed. Sometimes, if the tumour in the prostate is particularly large, a combination of radiotherapy and hormone treatment continuing after the radiotherapy has finished is recommended.

ADVANCED PROSTATIC CANCER

Unfortunately, when tests are done after cancer has been diagnosed, they often show that it is too advanced to be permanently cured by surgery or radiotherapy. Also, sometimes after initially successful treatment with surgery or radiotherapy, tests show that the cancer has recurred. However, this is far from being a hopeless situation. In the first place, the tumour may only be slow growing and elderly men with the disease may not have their lives shortened because of it. However, when prostatic cancer is more active, there is much that can be done to relieve symptoms and to slow its growth.

In addition to the usual prostatic symptoms, advanced prostatic cancer can cause backache (probably the most common effect) or pain in other bones, general ill-health with loss of weight, anaemia and other problems. Weakening of the bones can result in fractures but this is

How Hormones Work

The growth of the prostate gland, and of the prostate cancer, is controlled by the male sex hormone testosterone, made in the testes.

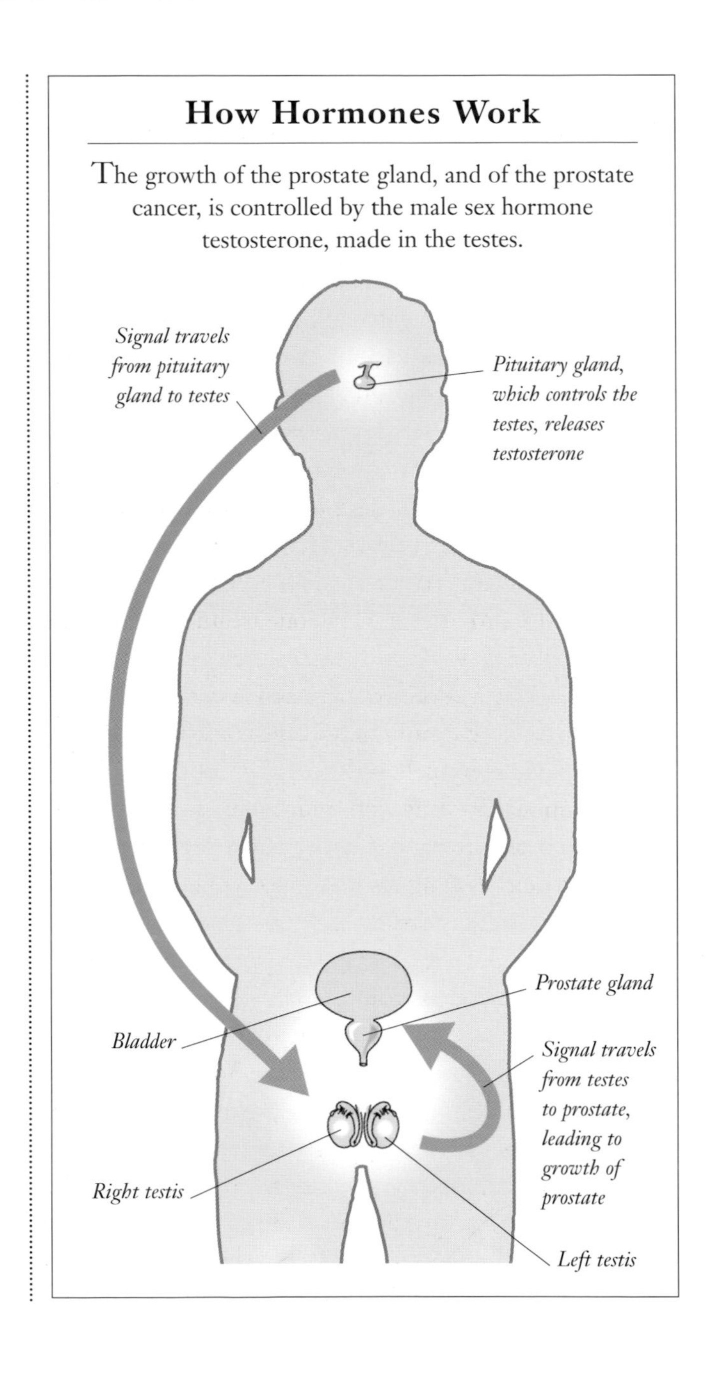

not common. Occasionally, cancer in the prostate can block the drainage of the kidneys. All these problems can improve, often almost completely, after treatment.

HORMONE TREATMENT

Just over 50 years ago, an American urologist called Charles Huggins found that if he removed the testicles from dogs with prostatic cancer, their cancer got smaller (regressed). He then treated some men by the same operation and some by giving them female hormones. He found that their disease responded in the same way. This was one of the earliest examples of an effective treatment for cancer that had spread beyond surgical cure. It was so important that Huggins was given the Nobel Prize for Medicine. Hormone treatment is still the most effective way of treating advanced cancer of the prostate, although there are now new ways of doing it.

The prostate will only grow and work if it receives normal amounts of male hormones (androgens). There are a number of different androgens and the most important is testosterone. Cancer of the prostate cannot grow without androgens, so depriving it of these hormones causes it to shrink and sometimes to disappear. Testosterone is produced from the testicles in response to a hormone that comes from a small gland at the base of the brain (the pituitary). As doctors and scientists have come to understand this, so new methods of hormone treatment have been developed. We now have much more choice than Dr. Huggins had back in the 1940s. The testicles can be prevented from producing the hormone, either by an operation to remove their functioning part (or sometimes the whole testicle is removed), or by drugs. Alternatively, there are drugs that act as a barrier between the tumour and the male hormones. These drugs prevent the androgens from stimulating the tumour cells without reducing the amount of androgens in the blood.

WHICH TREATMENT IS BEST?

Generally speaking, the effect of these different treatments on the tumour is the same. The choice between treatments is made on the basis of how they are administered and of their possible side-effects. Also, if one treatment does not suit an individual patient, it can be changed.

As with deciding between surgery and radiotherapy for early cancer, the patient may well be asked his opinion, and therefore it is useful here to give a little more information about the possibilities. As far as the patient is concerned, he can have:

- An operation that gets the whole thing over with so he no longer has to worry about taking treatment.
- An injection once a month or three monthly.
- Tablets.

As the hormone or drug treatments only work while they are being given, injections or tablets have to be taken indefinitely.

SURGERY AND INJECTIONS

The usual operation to reduce male hormone levels is called a subcapsular orchiectomy and involves making a cut into each of the testicles and removing the active tissue from the inside so that they no longer produce testosterone. Occasionally removal of the whole testicle might be recommended. The injections are of a type of drug called luteinising hormone releasing-hormone

(LHRH) analogue – for example, goserelin (Zoladex), leuprorelin (Prostap SR) or triptorelin (De-capeptyl sr). These injections stop the testicles producing testosterone and the effects are very similar to the operation. Goserelin and leuprorelin are now available as an injection that needs to be given only once every three months. Other three-monthly injections are being developed. A drug of a similar type called buserelin (Suprecur) is taken as a form of snuff into the nose, although this is not used much for treating cancer of the prostate.

Whether the treatment is an operation or a monthly injection, the level of male hormone is reduced and most men find that, as a result, their sexual activity – both their desire for sex and their ability to have an erection – is lost. Occasionally this does not happen, for reasons that are not understood; this should be thought of as a bonus and does not mean that treatment will not be effective.

Hot flushes, very similar to the condition experienced by women after the menopause, are another problem. These consist of feeling hot, or of attacks of sweating. Although fairly common, most men are only mildly affected and the condition tends to improve. If hot flushes are more severe, treatment is available. It is important to realise that they are a side-effect of the treatment – some men worry that hot flushes might be a sign that the cancer is advancing.

The effect of the operation on the testicles is to reduce their size, but the injection treatment also causes shrinkage. The testicles are associated with masculinity and it is natural to feel that this type of treatment involves 'castration'. However, most men with advanced prostatic cancer feel so much better as the treatment starts to work that this does not usually worry them too much.

PROS AND CONS OF BOTH TREATMENTS

Although the operation and the injections have very similar effects in the long run, there are differences between them at the time the treatment is started. Orchiectomy is only a fairly minor operation, but it does mean going into hospital, usually requires a general anaesthetic and is painful for several days. Minor complications such as bruising or swelling, or wound infection are not unusual. The operation works straight away and sometimes the symptoms are better as soon as the patient wakes up from the anaesthetic. The injections work more slowly and in fact during the first few weeks of treatment they actually cause an increase in the amount of testosterone. This could make the cancer grow a little and often for this reason tablets of another type of hormone treatment are also given for a few weeks, starting several days before the first injection.

TABLETS

Tablets may be prescribed because the patient prefers this type of medicine. If the patient really wishes to avoid the loss of sexual function, there is a type of drug called an antiandrogen that prevents the action of the testosterone on the tumour without reducing its level in the blood, and this can preserve sexual function. Available at the moment are flutamide (Drogenil) and nilutamide (Anandrone). Unfortunately, they tend to have more side effects, including gastrointestinal upset. A newly introduced drug called bicalutamide (Casodex) may have less side-effects, but at present can only be used with other drugs (see below).

Another drug called cyproterone acetate (Cyprostat) is also quite frequently prescribed. As well as blocking the effects of testosterone on the prostate, because it is similar to a type of female hormone, cyproterone acetate also reduces testosterone levels. Until recently, six tablets had to be taken each day but now a larger tablet is available.

Very rarely, it can cause damage to the liver and, as with all these treatments, must be carefully supervised.

At one time female oestrogen hormones such as stilboestrol were use a lot to treat cancer of the prostate. However, these drugs cause swelling of the breasts, but perhaps more importantly can have serious effects on the heart. Although female hormones can be used safely in very small doses, most men who are treated with tablets are given one of the other types of drug.

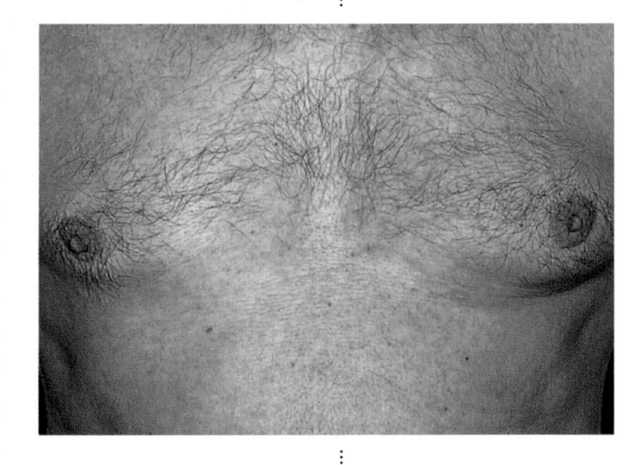

SWOLLEN BREASTS
One of the side-effects of female oestrogen treatment for prostate cancer is swollen breasts, so these drugs are no longer prescribed in large doses.

There are other ways of giving hormone treatment and newer and possibly better ones are being developed. However, the treatments mentioned here are the most common ones.

Recently it was found that a greater reduction of male hormone is possible by using a combination of drugs. This is because the adrenal glands also make male hormones and are not affected by orchiectomy or by LHRH analogues. Whether this more intense treatment actually improves results has been much debated by specialists. There is some evidence that it does, at least in some circumstances, and some patients receive it. Unfortunately, it is more complicated and can cause more side-effects.

OTHER TREATMENTS

If the cancer has spread to bone and is causing pain, radiotherapy can be very effective and usually works quickly. Sometimes a course of treatments – usually 10 – is given, on an outpatient or inpatient basis. Sometimes only a single treatment is necessary. Usually there are few problems but, depending where the painful area is, a mild stomach or bowel upset might occur.

A new method of giving radiotherapy to the bone is to use a radioactive substance called strontium-89. This selects the parts of the bone where the cancer is and gives it very intense but localised and safe radiation. It is given on an outpatient basis by a simple injection, so is very easy, although some simple precautions about radiation are needed for a day or two. Note that it was strontium-90 that used to cause all the concern about radioactive fallout – strontium-89 is a completely different type of strontium as far as its radiation is concerned, and does not have the same harmful effects.

KEY POINTS

- Prostatic cancer may be treated by surgery, radiotherapy or hormone therapy.
- Removing the whole prostate (radical prostatectomy) is possible when the cancer is only inside the prostate.
- Radiotherapy is an alternative to radical prostatectomy and can treat a tumour too advanced for surgery.
- Hormone treatment has proved useful for advanced prostatic disease.

Prostatitis

Prostatitis, or inflammation of the prostate, is generally the result of an urinary tract infection that has spread to the prostate. It is usually treated with antibiotics.

ACUTE PROSTATITIS

Inflammation of the prostate can occur at almost any age. It is often due to infection. Although cystitis – an infection of the urine causing burning and frequency – is more commonly a disease that affects women, these symptoms can occur in men. Such symptoms may be caused by an infection of the prostate called acute prostatitis. This may cause a high temperature and make the patient feel very unwell. In an older man who also has BPH, any prostate symptoms might become worse and prostatitis can sometimes cause retention of urine.

Sometimes an infection of the testicle called epididymitis complicates prostatitis and the symptoms from this might overshadow those from the prostate itself. As with simple cystitis, it is treated with antibiotics. However, the prostate does not take up antibiotics very well and some antibiotics do not work properly inside the prostate. If an infection of the prostate is suspected, the most likely type of antibiotic to be used is called a quinolone – examples

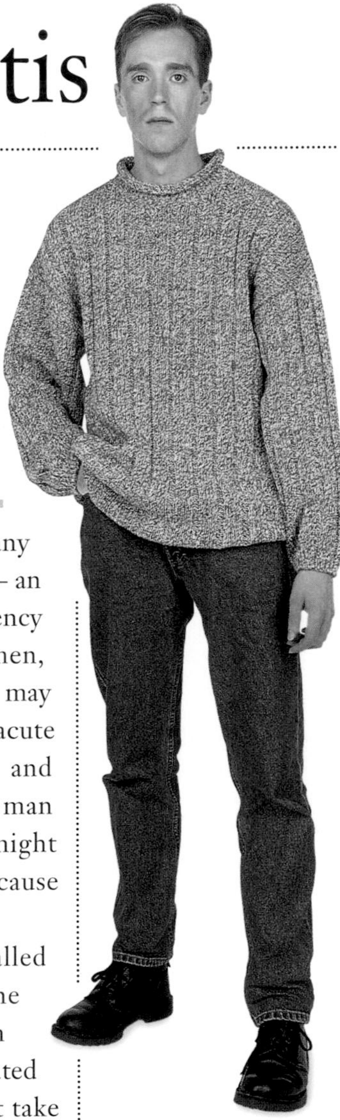

YOUNG MEN, TOO
Infection of the prostate can affect men of all ages, and can give rise to symptoms associated with cystitis.

are ciprofloxacin (Ciproxin), ofloxacin (Tarivid), norfloxacin (Utinor). It is important that the antibiotic is used for long enough to get rid of the infection completely. This usually means several weeks of treatment. It is important that the full course of antibiotics is taken, even if the symptoms have gone completely, to prevent the infection flaring up again.

Taking plenty of fluids and resting is important while the symptoms are bad. Avoiding sex is probably wise but most patients won't feel like it anyway while the symptoms are bad! Afterwards, frequent sex might help, as every time a climax is reached the fluid from the prostate may flush out any remaining infection. Rarely an abscess might develop. This is treated by letting out the pus by an operation very similar to a TURP.

CHRONIC PROSTATITIS

This can lead to occasional flare-ups of cystitis symptoms or cause more chronic pain. Such pain occurs in the lower abdomen, the testicles, between the legs or even in the back passage. Chronic prostatitis can be very difficult to diagnose, as the symptoms it produces can be due to all sorts of conditions, not necessarily involving the prostate. If they are caused by prostatitis, the prostate may be tender on examination. The doctor may try to grow bacteria from the prostatic fluid, which can be obtained by massaging the prostate or by getting a sample of semen.

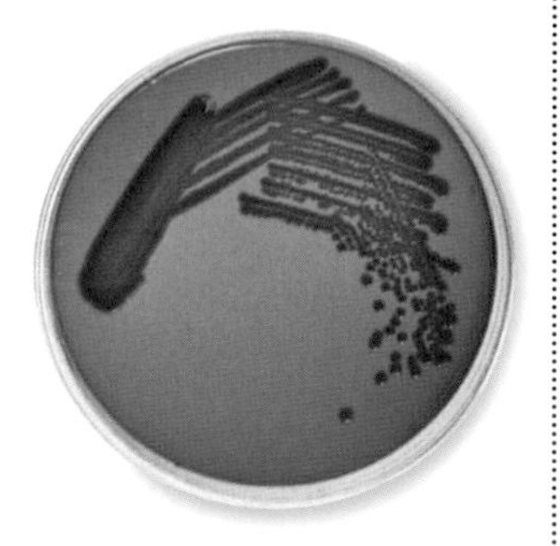

MAKING A DIAGNOSIS
Culturing a sample of fluid from the prostate for bacteria will confirm a diagnosis of prostatitis.

Sometimes the prostate is inflamed, but does not seem to be infected by bacteria. The cause of this type of prostatitis is not really understood but the symptoms are sometimes helped by anti-inflammatory drugs such as ibuprofen (Brufen, Nurofen) or indomethacin (Indocid) – although many similar drugs might be used.

PROSTATODYNIA

Similar symptoms to those of prostatitis are caused by a condition called prostatodynia. This probably results from spasm of the muscle in the prostate and certainly many men who suffer from it are helped by the same alpha-blocker drugs that are used in BPH (see p.45).

Conditions caused by muscle spasm are often aggravated by anxiety and stress, and some men do find that their symptoms are likely to occur if, for example, they are having a difficult time at work. Worry about the condition itself can also make it worse. In such cases it is very helpful to have the prostate checked out and be reassured that there is nothing else wrong with it. It is very unusual for pain in the prostate to be caused by cancer.

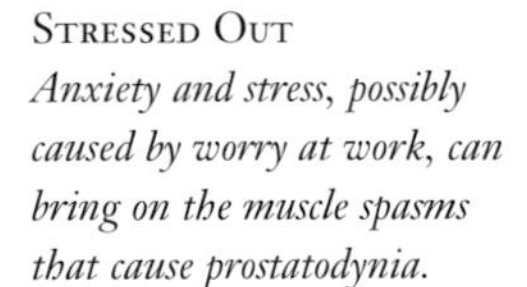

STRESSED OUT
Anxiety and stress, possibly caused by worry at work, can bring on the muscle spasms that cause prostatodynia.

OTHER CAUSES OF PROSTATITIS

Remember that prostatitis can be very difficult to diagnose and its symptoms are not very specific. You might be referred to a urologist to see if you have prostatitis. If he finds nothing wrong you may be referred to another specialist to make sure that there is no other cause of your symptoms.

KEY POINTS

- Inflammation of the prostate (prostatitis) may be caused by infection.
- Treatment is usually with antibiotics.

Improving the treatment

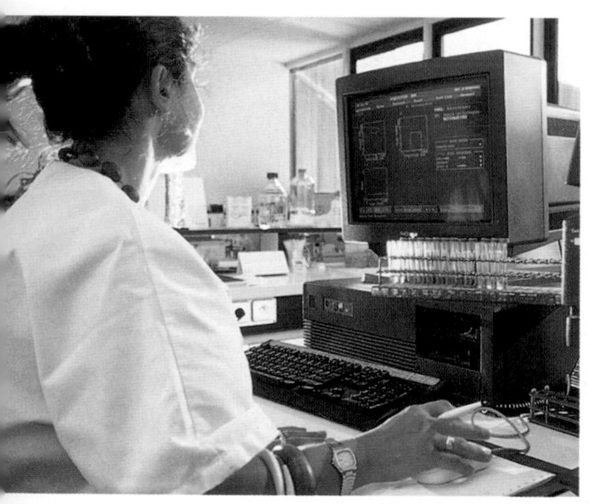

DRUGS RESEARCH
The search for new and effective drugs for treatment of prostate disorders holds out the long-term hope that operations may one day be unnecessary.

This book makes it clear that there have been many new developments in managing prostate disorders. As BPH is so common, it would be a major step forward in improving men's health if we could find a way of preventing it.

In fact this may already be possible. From the way it works, the new prostate drug, finasteride, might be better at preventing BPH than treating it once it has occurred. Unfortunately, all men would have to start taking it when they reach 40 and continue every day for the rest of their lives. For a disease that in most cases is a nuisance rather than life-threatening, this is not practical, nor could our over-stretched National Health Service afford it.

As new, more effective drugs are found and technology such as thermotherapy and laser devices is improved, the day may come when TURP and other 'old-fashioned' prostate operations are no longer done – probably not in your lifetime, or that of most urologists.

Cancer of the prostate is a very important disease. If treatments were simpler and easier than removing the prostate or radiotherapy, it would be much more feasible to tackle it by screening to look for early disease. We are beginning to know a little more about its causes, and might find ways of preventing it. Trials of drugs that could stop cancer of the prostate developing are being carried out in America.

CLINICAL TRIALS

Many new methods of treatment for both BPH and cancer are being tried at present. Such treatments can only be tested with the help of people with the disease. These are called clinical trials and are an essential part of showing that a new treatment really does work and that it is safe.

If you have a prostate condition you might be asked to take part in a clinical trial. Usually, this will be for a treatment that has already been extensively tested, so is almost certainly safe and there is a good chance it will be helpful. Indeed, sometimes being in a clinical trial is the only way to be treated with a promising new drug.

Most clinical trials are of a type known as double-blind randomised studies. These either compare two different treatments or compare one treatment against an inactive dummy treatment, which is

HELPING IN TRIALS
In clinical trials, you may either be given an active treatment or a placebo. Neither you nor the doctor will know which you are being given.

called a placebo. The comparison is only worthwhile if the treatment that each patient takes is chosen by chance, or randomisation. So that the interpretation of the results is done fairly, neither the patients nor the doctors running the trial know which of the treatments each patient is taking (although if a patient really needs to know, their type of treatment can easily be found out).

WHY IS A PLACEBO NECESSARY?

Simply seeing a doctor tends to make you feel better. This placebo effect is seen a lot in trials in BPH. This may be because the attention the patients receive makes them less bothered about their disease, and one result of this is that the muscle in the prostate relaxes. Patients receiving only inactive placebo may notice fewer symptoms, but their flow rate may also improve, so it is very important to compare drugs with a placebo to make sure that it really is the drug that is making things better.

If you do take part in a trial, you will certainly receive a lot of attention and many patients appreciate this. On the other hand it does also mean attending the hospital much more often, and some people find this difficult. The main disadvantage in most trials is that you have to have lot of blood samples taken – if you cannot stand needles, trials are not for you.

Before a trial is allowed to take place in any hospital, it will have been carefully considered by either a regional or the hospital's own Ethical Committee to make sure that it is safe and sensible. You will be given a very full explanation both verbally by a doctor and in writing, and it will be entirely your choice whether you take part. You should not take part simply to please the doctor. No one will object if you do not accept an invitation to join a trial and you will still get all the treatment you need. However, most patients who take part in trials quite enjoy it and usually find that they benefit from the treatment.

WHO WILL TREAT YOU?

Many diseases are treated by both hospital specialists and GPs, sometimes jointly. Patients with diabetes and high blood pressure will be familiar with this. Until recently, the only real treatment for BPH, the most common disease of the prostate, was an operation. This meant referral to a hospital urologist and it was not worthwhile for GPs to get too involved – there were too many other calls on their time. Unless the GP decided the problem was so mild that no treatment was going to be needed, a referral to a urologist was obviously the best thing for the patient, and even now most men with prostate problems will be seen and investigated in a urology clinic.

However, the treatment of prostate disorders has changed now that there are drugs that can be prescribed for BPH. Men with prostate symptoms are now less tolerant of their symptoms. People are living longer so there are far more men who are old enough to have prostate trouble than there used to be. Moreover, the Government has changed the way the Health Service works, so that there are benefits to GPs in doing more themselves and community care is being encouraged.

Milder forms of BPH can be managed with drugs, so it is no longer absolutely necessary for a surgical specialist such as a urologist to treat every patient. However, it is important that the patient and his prostate are carefully looked at before starting treatment, both to make sure that drugs are the correct choice and also to rule out cancer or other serious conditions that do need to be treated by a urologist.

Some GPs have become very enthusiastic about this, and a few health centres are now equipped with urine flow machines so that most of the important tests can be done by the GP. More often, the GP wants to know about the tests but cannot do them all. Many hospitals are setting up 'Open Access BPH Clinics' where the patient can go for the tests without having to be seen by a consultant urologist. Quite a few of these clinics are staffed by specially trained nurses – although a doctor is usually available, especially to do the rectal examination of the prostate.

The results of the tests are sent to the GP, but will also be looked at in the hospital and usually some advice is given. Any evidence of cancer will be picked up and the patient would then be seen promptly by the urologist in charge of the clinic.

This system has many advantages for the patient.

- He will almost certainly be seen quicker – most clinics offer appointments within a month or less.
- In a clinic where only men with prostate disease are seen, everything will be done more efficiently.
- The staff are all knowledgeable about the particular problem and may have more time to give information and to answer questions.
- Many men are more comfortable having a somewhat embarrassing problem dealt with in close consultation with their GP, whom they may have known for years, than they are seeing a strange hospital specialist.

This is a new development in health care, and many Open Access Clinics have been set up within the past few years. It is difficult to predict the future, but large health centres could start to run their own clinics, either with a visiting hospital urologist or, perhaps, with one of the partners in the practice, specialising, not only in managing BPH, but other urinary diseases. Patients should be reassured that these changes can only improve the care of men with BPH and reflect the increased awareness of this condition in recent years.

KEY POINTS

- Determined efforts are being made to find better treatments for prostate disorders.
- Clinical trials are an essential to show that a treatment really does work and is safe.

Case histories

Case History 1: **PROSTATE CANCER**

Mr. Alan James, a man of 68, had had a transurethral resection (TURP) for Benign Prostatic Hyperplasia (BPH) some years earlier. He developed further symptoms. When Mr. James was examined, his prostate was small but was very hard, and some tissue taken from it showed cancer. It was planned to give radiotherapy to the prostate, but a bone scan showed that there were a few small areas of cancer in the spine. These were causing no symptoms and as Mr. James was well, and his prostate was no longer giving him trouble, he decided that he would prefer not to be treated. He knew that it was important to be closely watched and he was seen by the urologist every few months and his PSA measured. Over the next 15 months, his PSA slowly started to rise, and his prostate symptoms came back. Although his bone scan had not altered, it was decided that he should have some hormone treatment. Because he did not fancy losing his potency, he was treated with flutamide. Mr. James' prostate symptoms improved and within three months, the PSA had become completely normal. All remained well for 18 months, when the PSA started to rise again. He was started on injections of an LHRH drug, and then the flutamide was stopped. He remains well and his PSA has fallen a little once more.

This tells us a lot about cancer of the prostate. Because cancer develops in the outer part of the prostate, having a TURP for BPH does not mean that cancer cannot develop later. Where the disease is detected at a fairly early stage, having a delay in treatment may not matter. This reduces the risk of side-effects, as also does choosing the right treatment for the patient – flutamide because he wanted to remain potent. Although the effect of hormone treatment is not permanent, changing treatment is sometimes helpful. Although Mr. James has been quite lucky, he has kept well for several years, showing that cancer of the prostate, even when it cannot be cured, can often be kept under control. Because treatment is effective, it is important to keep outpatient appointments, especially if treatment has been deferred. Note the amount of choice Mr. James had about his treatment.

Case History 2: **RETENTION OF URINE**

Mr. Robert Cohen, aged 90, attended a urologist because he was having trouble passing his urine. His prostate felt quite large. M.r Cohen's PSA was measured and was almost 40 (10 times the normal level). This is usually considered to mean that there is definitely cancer in the prostate. As he was so old and not very fit, the best treatment was difficult to decide, but meanwhile he came into hospital with retention of urine and needed a catheter. As Mr. Cohen could not pass urine when the catheter was removed, it was decided he should have an operation and, because the prostate was so large, it had to be taken out at an open operation. The prostate was found to weigh 350 grams (over 12 oz). As most enlarged prostates are less than 40–50 grams (1.5–1.8 oz), this was very large indeed. The pathology examination confirmed it to be BPH with no evidence of cancer.

An open operation, although a bit old fashioned, is still the best way to deal with a very large prostate. In BPH, the level of PSA depends on the size of the gland. If the gland is unusually large, like Mr. Cohen, the PSA will also be much higher than would be expected for BPH. This emphasises the problems of using PSA to diagnose cancer.

Case History 3: **BLADDER TUMOUR**

Mr. Ray Phillips, aged 60, was admitted for a prostate operation for which he had been waiting for a few months. Two days before admission, for the first time ever, he noticed some blood in his urine. Although the bleeding had stopped, the urologist did a careful cystoscopy examination of the bladder before starting the actual TURP and found a small tumour in the lining of the bladder, which was simple to remove at the same time.

It is never safe to assume bleeding is from the prostate, even if the prostate is causing other symptoms. If another cause is found, it is most often a bladder tumour. Although there is no connection between bladder tumours and BPH, it is very common, so a lot of men with bladder tumours will also have BPH.

Case History 4: **URETHRAL STRICTURE**

Mr. Sam Goldstein, a man of 65, complained of difficulty passing urine about six months after a heart operation (a coronary artery by-pass graft performed for angina). His prostate was enlarged, and he was referred to a urologist to see if a prostate operation was needed. The urologist did a cystoscopy and found a stricture in the urethra. This was cut open by a small operation called a urethrotomy, which is done with an instrument similar to that used to do a TURP. This completely cured Mr. Goldstein's symptoms, even though his prostate was enlarged.

Other things can cause prostate-type symptoms, so even if the prostate feels enlarged it may not be the cause of trouble. A catheter is used during heart operations to help check that enough urine is coming. The urologist knew that this can occasionally cause a urethral stricture and advised a cystoscopy examination.

Case History 5: **SUBMEATAL STRICTURE**

Two months after a TURP, Mr. Andrew Roberts felt that his symptoms were coming back and noticed that his urine was spraying as it left the tip of his penis. He went back to the urologist who diagnosed a short stricture just behind the external urinary opening. This was gently stretched with some metal dilators, and after this had been done a few times. Mr. Roberts had no more trouble.

Called a submeatal stricture, this is not unusual after a TURP and is easily treated. Do not despair if all is not going completely smoothly after a prostate operation. Many of the problems are simple to put right.

Case History 6: **RAISED PSA**

Having had mild prostate symptoms for a few years, 70 year-old Mr. John Pearson saw his GP because he had suddenly become worse. A blood test was done, and Mr. Pearson's PSA was 10 – significantly raised, although not very high. It suggested the possibility of cancer. He saw a urologist three weeks later, who examined the prostate, which felt benign, and retested the PSA, which was 7. This was reassuring and, two months later, not only had the PSA returned to normal but the patient's symptoms had also resolved and nothing more needed to be done.

Mr. Pearson clearly had some sudden event affecting his prostate, perhaps a mild infection, or a little internal bleeding sufficient to cause bruising or swelling without external evidence of blood. Sometimes a large prostate can lose part of its blood supply and the 'dead' area causes temporary swelling. Some urologists believe this is what happens to men who suddenly get retention when they have had no previous trouble. When something like this happens, PSA is released into the blood and increases the amount measured.

Just because a single PSA measurement is high, it is wrong to jump to conclusions about cancer. Indeed, BPH alone could cause the level of PSA found at first in Mr. Pearson.

Case History 7: **ACUTE PROSTATITIS**

Mr. William Hadley, a 58 year-old man, returned from a dinner party. When Mr. Hadley passed urine, he had severe burning pain and noticed his urine stream was poor. He had a sudden shivering attack. A few hours later Mr. Hadley's temperature was 39°C. He called his doctor who started Mr. Hadley on antibiotics. He felt better, but continued to have difficulty passing urine. When it almost completely stopped, he saw a urologist who advised immediate admission to hospital. His prostate was hard but also tender. His PSA was 25 (six times normal). A catheter was passed and the antibiotics continued. After a few days he was able to pass urine when the catheter was removed, but still with some difficulty. He continued to take antibiotics. His symptoms gradually improved and his PSA fell, although it was two months before it was back to normal. When he had completely recovered, his prostate felt soft and benign once more, but his urine flow rate was still well below normal.

Mr. Hadley had severe acute prostatitis. Despite not being aware of it, the fact that his flow rate on recovery was reduced probably means that he already had some obstruction from his prostate and the swelling from the prostatitis pushed him into retention. Acute prostatitis can make the prostate feel hard and can cause very high levels of PSA – indeed it may be best not to measure it in this situation. The raised PSA takes a long time to recover. Mr. Hadley took antibiotics for six weeks – stopping the treatment for prostatitis too soon can lead to relapse. It does seem that prostatitis is sometimes precipitated by drinking alcohol.

Questions and answers

Why do benign prostatic hyperplasia (BPH) and cancer of the prostate only occur in older men?
Some growth of the prostate probably occurs throughout adult life, under the influence of male hormones. About the age of 50, changes take place in the way the body produces and deals with male hormones, and this seems to cause the more rapid growth that is BPH. These hormone changes might influence cancer of the prostate, but many other types of cancer also occur more commonly in older people. This is probably because whatever causes the cancer takes many years to have an effect.

Why doesn't everybody with BPH get symptoms from it?
We do not quite understand this. Certainly a small prostate can cause very bad symptoms, while men with huge prostates can have virtually no trouble. It probably depends partly on just how the prostate squeezes the urethra and how well the bladder can cope with any obstruction. Anyway, it is all relative. Probably there are very few elderly men who are not a little bit affected, but many have symptoms so mild and that develop so slowly that they do not really notice them.

Does frequent sex make you more likely to have prostatic disease?
No, nor does it seem to protect against it. A study of abstinents showed that they were just as likely to get cancer of the prostate as the rest of us.

Can disease from the prostate cause illness in sexual partners?
No. BPH is specific to the prostate so it cannot occur in females, and in any case it is not caused by anything that could be transmitted in this way. The same applies to prostatic cancer. Although it is possible for the prostate to be affected by sexually transmitted infections, this is unusual, and prostatitis carries no risk to the patient's partner, nor is it caught by sexual contact.

I sometimes see blood in my semen – is this a sign of prostate disease?
Blood in the semen is quite common, although for obvious reasons it might not always be noticed. Unlike blood in the urine, it is rarely a sign of serious illness. It can be compared to a nose bleed. Like nose bleeds, it can sometimes occur repeatedly for a short period of time then settles down. Just as most nose bleeds are harmless, so is blood in the semen. Very rarely, they can both be a sign of a disease affecting the blood, or something like high blood pressure, or can result from some local disease that causes bleeding.

Occasionally, blood in the semen is associated with small stones in the prostate, and it can sometimes complicate prostatitis. Although BPH and prostate cancer can cause bleeding, this is usually seen in the urine. Blood in the semen is not something to worry about it but, especially if it occurs repeatedly, it is sensible to have it checked out.

Can I do anything to reduce the risk of prostate disease?
Probably not. However, if you have a bit of trouble, it is possible to stop it getting worse by being sensible. It is important to drink enough. Spread your drinking evenly through the day – if you are liable to wake at night cut down a little in the evening and do not drink a lot of tea, coffee or beer just before going to bed. Avoid hanging on too long, and make a point of passing urine regularly at comfortable intervals. On the other hand, if you do find you are getting a bit of frequency, do not let it take over – it is easy to get into the habit of passing urine more often than you really need to, and this just makes things worse.

I've just had prostatitis. Does this mean I'm likely to get prostate trouble when I'm an old man?
Not really. Prostatitis does not cause either BPH or cancer. Of course, prostate trouble is common, so you might be going to get it anyway.

I sometimes have pain in my testicles. Is this due to prostate disease?
Pain in the testicles is a very common symptom. Usually no cause can be found for it and it settles down without treatment. At the best of times, the testicles are a bit sensitive, and sometimes this sensitivity seems to increase for a while for some reason. Discomfort occurs from time to time in men who have had vasectomy operations. Because the tubes from the testicles go into the prostate, it is possible for infection to spread down them. Very painful swelling of the

epididymus, which is attached to the back of the testicle, called epididymitis, sometimes occurs in men with BPH or during an attack of prostatitis. If a hard lump is felt in the testicle itself it could be a tumour and should be reported to your doctor straight away.

My father died from cancer of the prostate. Is the same thing likely to happen to me?

Not necessarily. However, there seems to be a type of prostatic cancer that runs in families. If two or more closely related members of your family have had prostatic cancer, especially when they were fairly young, it is probably worth having your prostate checked from time to time once you get to 45 or 50.

I have heard that there is a herbal treatment I can buy at the chemist – wouldn't this be better than having an operation or taking drugs?

There are very many herbal and plant treatments said to help prostate disease. Although not used very much in the UK, they are very popular in some European countries. In fact, the Worldwide Fund for Nature is now worried because a species of tree has almost been wiped out because its bark is thought to be an effective treatment for BPH.

Most of these treatments have not been properly tested. If they work it may just be a 'placebo effect' (see p.81). However, there is no reason why plants should not make substances that work a bit like the drugs prescribed for BPH.

However, these plant substances could have just as many side-effects, if not more, than the properly prescribed drugs, so may not be any 'safer'. If you want to try tablets to help your prostate, you should ask your doctor about one of the drugs described on p.44. They have been proved to work and to be safe.

I've been referred for some prostate tests in a clinic that is run by a nurse. I've heard she might do the rectal examination of my prostate. Surely this is something only a doctor should do?

Specially trained nurses are being employed more and more to do the tests needed to check the prostate. As they specialise, they become very good at it. Almost everything else that is done in a clinic of this type is done by nurses in other areas. To have a doctor available to do the rectal examination is a bit wasteful of resources. If a nurse does examine the prostate (and this is still quite unusual), it will only be after she or he has been very well trained – just as she or he would be before being entrusted with, for example, measuring blood pressure. The nurse will do it many times a week, whereas doctors who do not work in urology departments may only need to do it occasionally. Although you might feel that a female nurse should not be doing this to a male patient, putting suppositories into the back passage is a very traditional nursing job that is not really that different.

I'm just 50. If I'm so likely to get prostate trouble could I have an operation now to prevent it?
No! A transurethral resection (TURP) only removes part of the prostate so you could still develop BPH or cancer some years later. Complications such as a urethral stricture might occur and be even more of a nuisance. Also, you would have retrograde ejaculation for the rest of your life.

Useful addresses

Prostate Cancer Charity
Du Cane Road
London W12 0NN
Helpline: (0181) 383 1948

Prostate Help Association
Langworth
Lincoln LN3 5DF

Better Prostate Health
PO Box 2846
London W6 9LW
Helpline: (0891) 667788

The Prostate Association
Stanley House
22 Paradise Street
Rugby CV21 3SZ

Prostate Research Campaign
36 The Drive
Northwood
Middlesex HA6 1HP

Send a 9" x 7" (23 x 18 cm) stamped addressed envelope for further information.

Index

Acknowledgements

PUBLISHER'S ACKNOWLEDGEMENTS

Dorling Kindersley would like to thank the following for their help and participation in this project:

Production Controller Michelle Thomas; **Consultancy** Dr. Sue Davidson; **Indexing** Indexing Specialists, Hove; **Administration** Christopher Gordon.

Illustrations: (p.11, p.12, p.13, p.19, p.24, p.41, front cover, bottom left) ©Philip Wilson; (p.68) Mark Roberts

Picture Research: Angela Anderson; **Picture Librarian:** Charlotte Oster.

PICTURE CREDITS

The publisher would like to thank the following for their kind permission to reproduce their photographs. Every effort has been made to trace the copyright holders. Dorling Kindersley apologises for any unintentional omissions and would be pleased, in any such cases, to add an acknowledgement in future editions.

APM Studios p.50, front cover, bottom centre; **Science Photo Library** p.17 (Alexander Tsiaras), p.22, p.20 (Michael Abbey), p.27 (Sue Ford), p.32 (CNR), p.37 (Mura Jerrican), p.54 (St. Bartholomew's Hospital), p.58 (Conor Caffrey), p.72 (Dr. P Marazzi), p.76 (Geoff Tompkinson), p.78 (BSIP LECA), p.79 (Geoff Tompkinson), front cover images: top left (Michael Abbey), top right (CNR), top centre (St. Bartholomew's Hospital), bottom right (CNRI)